STOP THE WORLD

SNAPSHOTS FROM A PANDEMIC

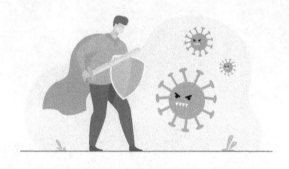

edited by

LISE MCCLENDON *with*

TAFFY CANNON • KATE FLORA • GARY PHILLIPS

THALIA

CONTENTS

PART III
STORIES FROM AROUND THE GLOBE

PART IV
A WRITER'S MIND

Most illustrations are by United Nations Covid-19 Response Creative Content artists. Thank you all.

Title page illustration designed by pch.vector / Freepik

Front cover illustration by Zoe Phoenix, age 8.

© 2020, Zoe Phoenix

Illustrations by Kate Hourihan

© 2020, Kate Hourihan

Photographs thanks to generous photographers on Unsplash

INTRODUCTION

2020 will go down as a year we are unlikely to forget. We have had many challenges this year, with more no doubt to come. But the COVID-19 pandemic that began at the end of 2019 and ravaged the world in 2020, killing countless people in every country, will be something we may want to forget. That was the genesis of this anthology. To record what we are likely to want to forget.

The idea came to me from two different sources. The first was a brainstorm I had early in 2019 for a worldwide happening on the same day, to simply share a meal with friends, family, neighbors, or strangers. To make a pot of pasta, some form of which is eaten everywhere, and share food with others. I called this idea 'One Night in the World' and envisioned it as a coming together, a communion, a uniting when we feel and see so much division everywhere.

This idea, like many of mine, sounded amazing but that I had little energy or expertise to make a reality. So, after scribbling a short page of notes, I set it aside and went back to writing. When I was cleaning up my computer desktop this spring (as one does while sheltering-in-place) I reread it and thought: what if instead I did an anthology about the pandemic? It's happening globally (unlike pasta night.) It would distract me from the horrors and give this awful time some purpose. Again, I did nothing, as is my natural reaction to my brainstorms.

Then I listened to a podcast with writer Cheryl Strayed ('Wild') where she discussed this unsettling time with her former writing professor. He said he recommended to his graduate students that they record their emotions and thoughts about this time because someday they would want to remember how it felt to be alive right now.

The universe, by way of that podcast, had slapped me awake. The professor was whispering in my ear: DO THE ANTHOLOGY. That very day, (before my native laziness set in again) I reached out to my writer friends, Gary Phillips, Kate Flora, and Taffy Cannon, who had previously co-written a hilarious crime novel (as Thalia Filbert) with Katy Munger and me. They immediately agreed to help.

This event, this horrible global pandemic, is obviously not humorous for patients nor the general public. The fear of disease, the lockdown, the economic woes were everywhere, as was the distraction of the news and whipsawing advice that wreaked havoc on many writers' focus and production, as evidenced by their essays here. Others found solace in the wry darkness of fiction. Some were called to poetry. The range and class of these pieces inspire me, and give me hope. I hope they do the same for you.

As the Earth spins on its axis, sometimes it seemingly stops and makes us look hard at our lives. We will move on, if we can, but for just this moment, take a look at these snapshots in time.

— Lise McClendon: June 2020

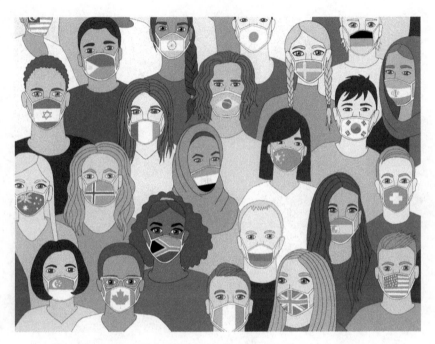

illustrations courtesy United Nations Covid-19 Response Creative Content artists

PART I

QUARANTINE LIFE

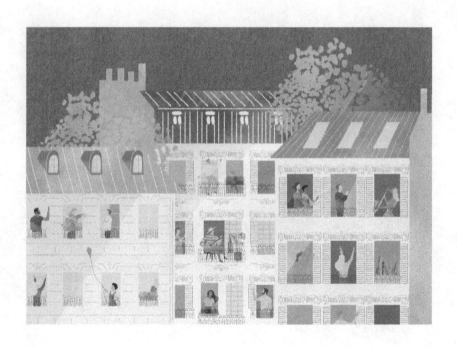

THE MARCH OF THE ANTS

BY DONNA MOORE

THE FIRST OF the ants came the day Lockdown started. Just a couple, determinedly trekking across the kitchen. They were mostly invisible, camouflaged against the dark grey floor tiles and counter tops. I spotted them, though, and the finger of fate descended on them firmly. And that was it, until a couple of days later, when there were one or two more of them. They experienced exactly the same fate as the earlier raiding party, but no lessons were learned from their non-return to the colony.

Over the next few days they route-marched their way across my kitchen. My eyes became accustomed to the tiniest flicker of movement and ants and breadcrumbs met the same vicious index finger. Ironically, the ants arrived at a time when my kitchen had never been cleaner. Every time Ewan and I came back inside from this new world where an invisible enemy lurked, we bleached every surface, to keep us virus free. In addition, enforced home confinement and reduced ability to concentrate on anything meant that the cupboards had never been cleaner. I Sleeping-With-The-Enemy-ed the cans and packets of food and enclosed bags of sugar and jars of honey in sealable bags, cutting off the ants' supply of hard drugs. My hands permanently smelled of bleach and the ants had nothing to feast on; yet still they came, blackly, relentlessly and optimistically.

I called to mind the few things I knew about ants: they can carry fifty times their own body weight, they survived the Ice Age, they're extremely clever. Yes, all very impressive, chaps, but I had the internet. What makes ants... I typed. Google suggested ...explode, ...mad, ...happy, ...so strong, ...go away. Don't get me wrong; in the normal way of things ants impress me. Their sense of community is amazing; they bury their dead; they're ruled by a woman (although the fact that after sex she doesn't eat for weeks is a tad strange, especially since ants have two stomachs); and they can become zombies. Yes, there's a lot to admire about ants. But not when they're in my house in ever-increasing numbers.

So I chose what makes ants go away. They don't like vinegar, I was assured. I filled a spray bottle with vinegar and water and sprayed all the skirting boards. I sprayed the counter tops, inside the cupboards, all over the cupboard doors. The trick, apparently, was to cover their tracks. They use their sense of smell to follow the pheromones of the ants who've boldly gone before. Google promised, but the ants continued to come. Turns out, the only beings in the house who were upset by the smell of vinegar were me and Ewan.

I rang my mum. "Talcum powder," she said. "Or flour. Anything powdery, they don't like to walk on it." Flour? This was Lockdown. Asking me to throw flour on the floor was like asking me to scatter diamonds and emeralds in front of the ants as though they were dignitaries visiting an exotic land. Come to think of it, it might have been easier to lay my hands on diamonds and emeralds when we hadn't managed to score any flour on fraught trips to the supermarket in the last four weeks. And, since there is neither a baby nor an eighty year-old woman in the house, we had no talcum powder. All I could rustle up was a jar of cinnamon and some dried ginger, which I sprinkled along what seemed to be the ants' preferred route.

Having worked out that their favorite times were dawn and dusk, I set the alarm for five in the morning. And I watched them as they marched across the no-man's land of cinnamon and ginger and carried on just as if their little feet weren't covered in spices. Still, at least the kitchen smelled reassuringly of cinnamon rolls and ginger-bread, rather than two-day old fish and chip suppers. Undaunted, I decided that no-man's land wasn't wide enough. I ordered two indus-trial-sized tins of Lily-of-the-Valley talcum powder and used up a whole tin sprinkling a two-inch strip around the whole kitchen and in the cupboards the ants seemed to like the most (alcohol, baking trays and teabags, incidentally). Everywhere was covered with ribbons of white powder. Had we been raided by the police, we would have been in trouble.

It worked. For a whole day. They were outsmarting me at every turn; it was as though they'd ordered hundreds of little pairs of boots from AntAmazon just to spite me. I held onto the fact that the kitchen now smelled like my grandmother. Comforting, but with added ants.

It was now week five of Lockdown, and week five of ants. I googled, and I bought. If anyone looks at my online shopping history, it will tell the story of a pandemic. 2010 all the way through to 2019: books. Books, books, books. 2020: face masks, hand sanitizer, chicken noodle soup mix, talcum powder, peppermint oil. Yes, peppermint oil was Google's latest suggestion.

I lined up some cotton wool balls and, like a scientist in her lab, I put a few drops of oil on each one. Eyes stinging, I put a couple of the cotton wool balls in every cupboard. Every time we opened one, an eye-watering waft of peppermint was released. What with the white talcum powder everywhere and the minty scent, Ewan took to calling the kitchen Donna's Festive Grotto. But it seemed to work. A few stray ants stumbling around in a peppermint-fueled stupor, too stoned to escape, were soon dispatched. OK, every cup of tea we drank and every sandwich we ate tasted like mint, but it was worth it for an ant-free home. I still checked every cupboard, dawn and dusk. On the fourth day, I saw two ants. I topped up the peppermint-infused cotton wool balls. The ants retreated, and for a week we've been ant-free.

"That wasn't like you," said Ewan. "The whole war on the ants thing. You took that way more seriously than you'd normally have done."

I think Ant-mageddon was a symbol of how I felt about COVID-19. I could see the ants, I could battle them, I could win against them. I can't see COVID-19 and the only thing I can do against the virus is to not do something. Not go out. My home is my safe place and when it's being invaded by ants it doesn't feel safe anymore. The ants are my visual representation of COVID-19. And now they're gone. But COVID-19 is still here. Lockdown is still here.

I miss the ants.

But my lawn is full of dandelions – cheery, brightly-colored, smiling demons of the underworld, with roots that go right down to the bowels of hell. Tomorrow I'll get out my dandelion-weeder and start on that lawn. I'll do battle with the dandelions and I'll win. I will win. We will win, just you see.

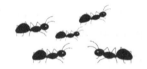

Donna Moore is the author of two humorous crime fiction novels and several short stories. She is currently undertaking a PhD in Creative Writing, writing three historical crime fiction novellas set between 1870 and 1920. In her day job she works with marginalized and vulnerable women to support them with their literacy. She is also co-host of the CrimeFest crime fiction convention. Oh, and she (reluctantly) knows far too much about ants. She lives in Scotland.

DON'T SNEEZE ON ME

BY JOHN REMBER

IT'S MAY. Forest Service trucks are making daily trips between the Stanley Ranger Station and the Sawtooth National Recreation Area Headquarters in Ketchum. Last summer there were a lot more, ten or twelve a day, usually with two or more passengers. Now, it's one person per vehicle, and only three or four go by from eight to five. We notice them when they pass. There's not much traffic since steelhead season closed.

Social distancing rules remain in place in Idaho. We are in Phase One of a four-phase plan to reopen Idaho's economy. Each phase is supposed to last two weeks, culminating in the opening of bars, theaters, and stadia, but Idaho's governor Brad Little has said that life won't return to normal until there's a cure or a vaccine, neither of which is guaranteed.

Churches and business offices can open if they observe strict social distancing and require personal protection equipment. Vulnerable people—the over 65s, the immunologically impaired, the obese, smokers, those with cardiovascular disease—are supposed to stay in their homes, if they have a home to stay in. People from outside of Idaho have been told to isolate themselves for two weeks before coming out to enjoy the freedoms of Phase Two, which include wider access to sunlight, well-spaced restaurant dining, and haircuts.

Governor Little, in his first term, has become a right-wing governor under attack from his right wing. Outraged demonstrators have protested outside of his office and home. One of our northern Idaho legislators has called him "Little Hitler" for his closure orders —but he has remained what he calls "data driven," which means he's listening to state health department epidemiologists, not Joseph Goebbels.

The reopening schedule depends on a continued decline in coronavirus cases. A super-spreading wedding reception, or a deliberate coronavirus party attended by people who want to get it over with, and we'll be back to loud bare-faced people lining up on Idaho's statehouse steps, waving AR-15s.

Vulnerability is best understood from the point of view of the vulnerable, and it's safe to say that if you make your living in the tourist economy, you're feeling as vulnerable as any fat 75-year-old with a two-pack-a-day habit and a heart transplant. Sawtooth Valley depends on tourists to live, and if they don't show up, or if they do show up and don't spend their money, our local businesspeople will face the end of their worlds.

About the only people who might be happy about these scenarios work for the Forest Service. The pandemic is an opportunity to further regulate Sawtooth Valley's tourist population. It's a job they appear to enjoy.

We could see masks on people floating the rivers, and mostly empty buses taking passengers back upriver. Those of us who grew up watching the Lone Ranger on after-school TV will do a double-take if we see groups of masked horseback riders, expecting them to shoot up the first saloon they come to. Guest lists of weddings will be vetted to ensure that no one will fly in from a coronavirus hot-spot. Old people will be permitted to watch at a safe distance, in groups of one.

You may find this picture disturbing and even horrifyingly totalitarian, but recognizable if you've been keeping up with the news.

Similar measures have evolved as the local economies across the country have dealt with coronavirus in their midst. In some cases, the virus has been more lethal to the economy than to human beings, although over time a dead economy can result in more dead people than the virus itself.

The armed demonstrators at the statehouse tend to fetishize camo clothing, and they pack weapons that they are more or less familiar with. They form public phalanxes in spite of official pleas to social distance. Appeals to their own safety or that of their grandparents only convince them that the real life-and-death matter is maintaining their own world view. They actively disrespect any government, even a respectable cloth-coat Republican state government like Idaho's. The federal government is their real enemy, and they know a federal uniform when they see it.

It's possible we'll get swarms of these people escaping locked-down cities and heading for the designated wildernesses that surround the valley. Wilderness is strongly connected with freedom in their minds, despite the fact that it's some of the most regulated real estate outside of downtown Manhattan. It's seen as a place where a bug-out bag and a rifle can allow you to live off the land for a year or two, despite another fact that if a few thousand like-minded people are out there with you, any wild game larger than a ground squirrel will be gone before winter.

Overwhelming unconscious forces can turn one person into a camo-wearing, open-carrying demonstrator waving a Don't Tread on Me banner. He'll sneeze in your face if you impinge on his personal freedom. Equally overwhelming unconscious forces can turn another person into a uniform-wearing federal officer who takes seriously his duty to make people behave. Sneezing in his face will be a felony, and he doesn't like felonies.

Self-awareness is not a big part of either process.

The pandemic has brought the deep impulse toward freedom and the equally deep impulse toward regulation to the surface of our lives. King Kong and Godzilla have emerged to do battle. Even if their avatars are puny and sometimes ridiculous humans, those humans are packing guns. If we're lucky, we locals will get to watch from a safe distance. Binoculars are recommended.

————

JOHN REMBER LIVES and writes in the Sawtooth Valley of Idaho. Recurring themes in his writing include the meaning of place, the impact of tourism on the West, and the fragility of industrial civilization. John's latest book, *A Hundred Little Pieces on the End of the World* was published in March of 2020 by the University of New Mexico Press.

3

THE DOWN-HOME CORONAVIRUS VICTORY GARDEN BLUES

BY TAFFY CANNON

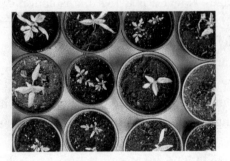

courtesy Markus Spiske

THE LAST THING I bought before I came home for good on March 12th was a Lemon Boy tomato plant. I had no idea that this would become the cornerstone of my impromptu Victory Garden.

I wasn't planning a vegetable garden at all. In San Diego we get fabulous produce year-round and I was pretty sure that would continue. I intended to spend a lot of garden time just hanging out this summer with my daughter and two-year-old granddaughter, who live an hour away.

A few days later the entire state of California shut down, as did that plan. I figured my husband and I could manage sequestration easily enough; we've both worked from home for a long time and know our boundaries and spaces. Indeed, my life turned out to be a lot like it was before I had a child, a book contract, or community responsibilities.

The garden, however, was different from the beginning.

When I do spring cleanup in my yard—a space filled with wondrous things but perpetually overplanted and overgrown—I don't normally water with my own tears. Through the first blurry weeks I continued the major cleanup I'd started after Christmas, and quietly passed the two-week mark then considered the longest incubation period.

I decided to grow as many vegetables as I possibly could.

Most of the places I dwell in my fantasy worlds are remote and isolated: islands, mountaintops, farms, lonely beaches, ranches, woodland cottages. Now I was living that isolation. My home and my garden became my sanctuary and my project. Apart from morning walks, I never left the property.

I set up parameters.

The Victory Garden would contain only what I already had or could grow from seed. No trips to the nursery. My herb garden was thriving, missing only annual basil and dill. I let last year's parsley and a forgotten scallion clump go to seed.

I would use seed from previous years and materials I already had, sometimes literally lying around. Unfortunately, I'd tossed much of my elderly seed stash last year when I planted a quixotic Rainbow Garden—Glass Gem Indian corn, with multi-colored collections of beets, radishes, pole beans, and Patty Pan squash.

I planted what seed remained in fifteen-gallon containers and ordered more from Renee's Garden, quick-maturing varieties. When they warned of shipping delays, I talked a Texas Hill Country friend into mailing me his own castoff seed, some literally retrieved from the trash. When I ordered from Renee's again later, my earlier selections had sold out.

I rarely sow directly into the ground, and hadn't started seedlings indoors for years. I was never very good at it anyway. Now I gave it my best shot and tried not to check my babies more than six or eight times a day.

Coddled seed grows very, very slowly. It was still too cold to plant these warm-weather crops outside, anyway. March crawled by and April meandered in.

But there was plenty to do in my increasingly manicured flower gardens. Spring flowers ignored the pandemic, and just walking out the back door soothed me. Pulling tens of thousands of weeds provided purpose as well as compost fodder. I refurbished a large vegetable bed that hadn't been used for years. I shored up and stained decaying trellises.

Time passed with none of the normal celebrations I love. St. Patrick's Day, my husband's birthday, Palm Sunday, Easter, my son-in-law's birthday, Mother's Day.

Everything scientific we learned about Covid-19 was confusing, contradictory, and likely to change tomorrow. Masks? No, then suddenly and dramatically yes, as sewing machines whirred from coast to coast. Government responses at national, state, and local levels often resembled overcrowded clown cars of the ill-informed. People were dying at terrifying rates in congested northeastern cities and the rural West thought it was all a leftist crock.

The West Coast curve was flattening, but testing remained a macabre joke. I pretended that my daughter and granddaughter lived in Nova Scotia, too far away for random weekend visits. Eventually I returned to the book due on September 1, a too-timely caregiving guide. Much later, I graduated from my comfort reads of Nancy Drew to Ross MacDonald, both anchored in earlier worlds.

I could escape everything in the garden.

With no traffic, skies blazed blue and bright, more so after rare heavy April rains. Most of the ambient noise of suburbia was gone, and in this neighborhood of older residents, life became deliciously quiet, save for bird songs. My mountaintop, my island, my woodland cottage.

I have never grown such pampered veggies: watered twice daily, thinned seedlings replanted elsewhere (successfully!). I cheated only once on my subsistence plan when I had my husband buy me dill and Supersweet 100 tomato plants at the nursery where I'd let him indulge a fuchsia-sale jones.

I decided to visit my own favorite nursery in June, even if I needed a Hazmat suit.

By mid-May, the Victory Garden was moving into its maintenance phase. When I finally got a functional soaker hose placed, my initial deep watering doubled the size of baby plants overnight and triggered a probable-leak warning from the water department. A baby bunny appeared. Days grew hot, and some of my seedling babies fried during their hardening stage. I stopped worrying about that because it was nearly June, when I'd mask up and head for the nursery.

Finished sweet peas moved to compost and tomatoes replaced them. Fruit appeared on the Blue Lake beans and Lemon Boy tomato and Patty Pan squash. Cucumbers climbed their supports and I snipped fresh dill into my morning eggs.

I passed the milestone I always miss at first: when I'm so busy with what's growing that I stop making inconsequential notes on my garden calendar. I always felt guilty about this until I read Thomas Jefferson's garden journals and discovered that he did the same thing.

We couldn't celebrate my daughter's sixth anniversary on May 31, because she was still in Nova Scotia.

But on June 1, I went to the nursery.

––––––

TAFFY CANNON IS the Agatha- and Macavity-nominated author of fifteen novels, mostly mysteries; an Academy Award-nominated short film; and SibCare: The Trip You Never Planned to Take. She lives in Southern California. www.TaffyCannon.com

4

SPRING WALKING IN THE YEAR OF QUARANTINE

BY TAMI HAALAND

In mid-May, I hike with my family through the local rimrocks, a network of cliffs and ponderosa pine, ravines and sagebrush, near our home in Billings, Montana. Despite the dry winter, spring flowers are abundant. We find larkspur couched in wormwood, wild sweet peas in colonies, shooting stars whose bright magenta blooms smell of jasmine, and along the trail prairie lilies clustered at ground level. It seems as if we can walk forever meeting only a few hikers or bicyclists along the way.

We are lucky, and we know it. I'm still employed, our grown sons are here, and one of them has planted a huge garden. We have fresh air, a house, a world of trails nearby.

The next day I follow a more urban route in calm and foggy air listening to Performance Today on American Public Media. The path takes me along baseball fields, past an irrigation ditch where Russian olive and cottonwoods compete for space, through a tunnel covered in children's colorful handprints, and to a park where it's possible to see miles into the western horizon. It has been one of the everyday walks that frames my work, creates some sort of pace and vision and fresh perspective during these many days at home. Snow or rain or sunshine, it has been a necessary part of the daily sanity, and only recently have I added music.

Now, walking in and of itself is not always enough to bring my mind back into focus. Too much worry, perhaps, or boredom or repetition have left me wanting more. A growing nostalgia for the way things used to be has helped me understand it may be years before we arrive at what we formerly considered normal movement about the world.

It's not that I'm terribly dispirited. I'm grateful every day, but when I add music to the emerging spring, something happens. A more surreal experience of place prevails. I am here and not here which corresponds to life in quarantine, the strangeness of inhabiting a new locked down world and disbelief that we've arrived here so quickly. On one of my walks, I admire flowering chokecherries in relation to Mahler's Symphony No. 7. Along a winding trail in the prairie, I listen to "Suite from Moby Dick" by Jake Heggie, arranged by Cristian Macelaru and played at the Aspen Music Festival the previous July. Suddenly the journey becomes epic, the coulees and hills become sea swells.

On another morning when the ominous rise in deaths from Covid-19 feels particularly heavy, David Lang's "Gravity" accompanies the last leg of my journey on a street between the wild rimrocks and suburban houses with their brilliant flowering crabapples. The scene is full of promise while Lang's delicate notes descend but, according to the composer, "never touch down." The slow runs seem to echo our current state, the mounting losses alongside anxious conversations about opening the world. The piece mirrors the sorrow, inescapable as gravity.

Lang's second piece, "Beyond Gravity," begins as I near home. It is livelier and more hopeful, the runs more buoyant, and it lifts my spirit as the body responds to these new rhythms.

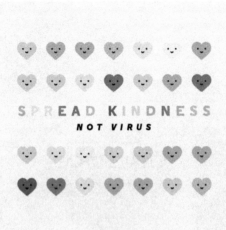

Ultimately, I have great faith in humanity. I hope we can see past the illusions of separation and understand we are part of an ecosystem where plants and creatures exist in relation, even because of relation to each other. But these lessons may continue to take hold slowly, and the human ego is so willing to counter with arguments for fierce independence and hierarchy. We are a mess, we humans, and we have potential, especially as this historic period reminds us, yet again, of our inevitable and intimate connection.

———

TAMI HAALAND IS the author of three poetry collections, most recently *What Does Not Return*. Her poems have appeared in many periodicals and anthologies, including, Consequence, The American Journal of Poetry, Ascent, The Ecopoetry Anthology, and Healing the Divide. Her work has also been featured on The Slowdown, The Writer's Almanac, Verse Daily, and American Life in Poetry. Haaland lives and teaches in Montana.

5

CARPE DIEM
BY CAITLIN ROTHER

MY PARTNER of eight years and I live apart together. Before the Rona, we spent three nights a week together, alternating between our two homes, and also enjoyed frequent out-of-town vacations. We've always enjoyed a good adventure, a new favorite restaurant or winery, or swimming out to the buoy. Creating and playing music together in an acoustic band brought us closer. We even considered doing a reality cooking show.

Then the Rona hit. With a history of inflammatory and respiratory issues, I obsessively read every news article about the novel coronavirus that incited inflammatory storms and turned lungs into glue. It took only one traumatic trip to the supermarket to keep me at home well before the shelter-in-place orders. As I absorbed every symptom and death statistic I could find, I wasn't going anywhere.

Not only am I a rule follower, but I also wanted to protect my future by staying away from those openly tempting fate and succumbing to Darwinism. While they chose to protest on Planet Delusion, I lived, cloistered, on the Planet of Natural Selection, where the smartest people survive.

My partner and I agree on politics, and we've been a couple long enough to learn how to keep conflicts down. Still, our views on risk assessment couldn't be more at odds.

He has a strong constitution and a high pain threshold. When he occasionally gets sick, he tries to ignore it. I fear illness because I've spent far too much of my life being sick or in pain. Early on, I bought masks even though we were told not to, because of the PPE shortage.

To me, "Don't go out or see anyone you don't live with" meant just that. But when most other people were sent home, he continued to go to work. He didn't have a choice, because he runs an essential business, but he also had no qualms about going to supermarkets or Home Depot, flying on airplanes, or renting cars.

I wanted to stay alive, even if it meant I couldn't see him for a while, so a couple weeks in, I told him it didn't feel safe to be around him. He lives half-time with his autistic teenager, who has OCD and likes to pick up and rearrange things all over my house. He also works with his millennial son, who shares the no-fear gene, and lives with several roommates. Too many risk factors for me.

So we entered the phase of nightly happy-hour video calls. Before, he'd spent so much time reading his phone that I often felt alone even when we were in the same room. But now we were talking again. Really talking. For hours.

After spending most days steeped in anxiety, these talks were a reprieve from my isolation and my escalating trepidation about venturing outside. Everything gave me the big, deep feels.

Then the arguing started.

"You're paranoid," he said. "I'm washing my hands."

"I don't feel safe," I replied. "I'm just following the health-safety guidelines that everyone is supposed to. I'm not making this up."

Still, I looked forward to these poignant, meaningful conversations, which we ended by bringing our puckered lips to the camera for a virtual kiss. I missed him. I cried. I loved him so much it hurt.

He brought me groceries so I didn't have to go out, but I couldn't let him come in anymore. So he'd drop off the bags, and we'd chat a few minutes.

"Are you ever going to the store again?" he asked.

As the weeks went on, he grew annoyed with not being allowed to come inside, so he delivered the groceries, then left.

"I'm tired of the 2-D love," he said one night.

We argued again about the precautions, the risks, the statistics, the rules. I feared I would lose him, but I was torn. I didn't want to die. There were so many unknowns. I needed more time.

We had a group video call with a friend who once worked in risk management and talked about the need to wear masks. When my partner started wearing one, along with everyone at his company, I started feeling a little safer.

So, after six weeks of isolation, I stepped out of my comfort zone and let him stay the night. But he had to follow my rules. After grocery shopping, he had to remove his clothes, shower, and put on fresh ones. He didn't normally take such precautions, but he did so for me. And he brought red roses.

It was a celebration. To see him, to hug, and to be touched. To drink wine, to laugh and eat dinner together. My heart swelled, then deflated, sad to see him go back to his life without me.

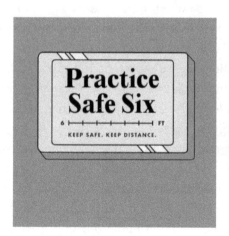

Another quarantine period followed, as I looked forward to our next rendezvous about three weeks later.

Shortly before he came over, however, he got a haircut, which was strictly forbidden at the time. When I noticed and said something, we were both so angry we didn't speak for almost an hour. He offered to go home. I said no. Stay.

So we took a silent walk, had some wine on the couch, and tried to relax.

"I thought I'd dress for the occasion," he said, re-emerging in the satin boxer shorts we'd bought when we first started dating. Following his lead, I put on the purple satin chemise he'd given me.

We put our vexation aside, kissed, and made love. I want to say we were back in our old comfortable bubble of intimacy, but it was different. Far more intense. Almost like goodbye sex.

Then it was time for the homemade sushi dinner we'd planned, bookended with hot sake and green tea mochi. Still wearing our silky lingerie, we took pandemic snapshots in my dimly lit kitchen, smiling and goofy, in what could be our last joyful moments, the best of what was left of our lives. Whatever and for however long that may be.

———

CAITLIN ROTHER IS the New York Times bestselling author or co-author of 13 books, including DEAD RECKONING, HUNTING CHARLES MANSON, and POISONED LOVE. Coming soon is DEATH ON OCEAN BOULEVARD: Inside the Coronado Mansion Case https://www.caitlinrother.com She lives in San Diego.

6

STICKY BUNS

BY JODY JAFFE

MY MAJOR ACCOMPLISHMENT during the time of Corona — other than not arguing with any of the Trumpers who live near me — was perfecting the sticky bun.

I've been making sticky buns for years, always to the oohs, aahs and glowing Instagram posts of important guests I want to keep luring back with my culinary wiles, — ie, my grown children. I made them for my second husband before he was my second husband. He might tell you that was a compelling reason to walk down the aisle and into a ready-made family of me and my two skeptical preadolescent sons.

That earlier version I made was good, it's hard to make a bad sticky bun. But it wasn't Sausalito Sweet Shop sublime. I ate that sticky bun 40 years ago on a trip with the man who would become my first husband and the father of those children who don't visit enough. The marriage soured and the years with him have dimmed, but the memory of that sticky bun still burns bright. They were a study in the perfect ratio of sweet amber goo to the soft cinnamon-laced cushion of puffy white bread, crowned by a blanket of caramelized pecans.

With so much time on my hands during lockdown, I spent more

minutes that I'd like to admit Googling "best sticky bun recipe" and reading through every comment. I could have embarked on any number of more important tasks, such as cleaning out my closet and giving away my pre-pregnancy clothes (children are 35 and 32) and at least one quarter of the 40-plus pairs of shoes I never wear.

But the pandemic scared me. Those two children live far away which meant I had no way of protecting them. My limbic brain was panicking. Short of getting on a plane to Thailand, where my older son was living, or driving seven hours north to the epicenter of the pandemic, where my younger son lives, I had to find a way to calm myself.

Who knew a little flour and yeast quiets the reptilian brain? There is something deeply soothing about watching and smelling dough rise. For me, this does not come from a return to the comfort of my childhood. My mother never baked anything in her life, let alone a loaf of bread. This is much much deeper. I'm talking epigenetically deep. This comfort comes from the shtetls of my past.

Studies show that bad memories pass down six generations in mice. Why not good memories? Where do they go anyway? To the land of missing Tupperware lids? Is whatever or whomever created us that cruel that she/he or it thought it would be funny to only pass along the bad shit? That would be too cruel for even the most vindictive of gods.

In my version of reality, the good memories burrow into our DNA along with the bad ones. So somewhere in Lithuania or Odessa or Kiev, my great great-great-great-great Bubbie always had dough rising, perfuming the air of our shack in the Pale.

Smell is a bullet train to the past. I lifted the cover of my rising sticky-bun dough and pressed my nose close. I inhaled deeply and everything felt like it would be all right. My son in Thailand would be safe, even though he is immuno-compromised. My other son in New York City would be safe, no "even thoughs," other than I am a worrier and he was not under my roof. My husband and I would make it through this pandemic alive, even though he is 73 and I am 67. Trump would not win the election.

All that from the yeasty smell of flour and water fermenting. A miracle of sorts, almost as good as the small cruse of oil that burned for eight days and eight nights when it was only supposed to last one day.

And my new version of the sticky bun? All that Googling paid off. They were, in fact, Sausalito Sweet Shop sublime.

———

JODY JAFFE IS the author of the Nattie Gold newspaper/horse show mysteries: "Horse of a Different Killer," "Chestnut Mare, Beware," and "In Colt Blood." She is also the co-author of the novels "Thief of Words," and "Shenandoah Summer." She and her husband, John Muncie, live on a farm in the Shenandoah Valley with eight horses.

SUBDIVISION QUARANTINE

BY ALLEN MORRIS JONES

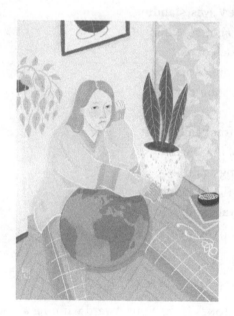

OUR LOVELY LITTLE HOUSES,
    appreciating predictably
    until now, tidy little

investments until now,
stand like ships set
to a larger purpose,
warships off to battle,
skirted in lawns, new
trees moored with posts
and twine, rising and falling
with the big rollers coming
in from the horizon,
the deep sea mountains
of water that lift us helplessly
up and drop us down again;
lift us up, drop us down;
six weeks now we've been
riding these waves, standing
with coffee at our kitchen
windows, each of us
set apart, families apart,
shoulder to shoulder
in the subdivision, waving
cheerfully, frantically from
the crests of the waves
before falling again
racing into the troughs
where we wait, and
wait.

———

ALLEN MORRIS JONES is the Spur Award-winning author of the novels *Sweeney on the Rocks, A Bloom of Bones,* and *Last Year's River,* as well as a nonfiction consideration of the ethics of hunting, *A Quiet Place of Violence,* and a children's book, *Montana for Kids: The Story of Our State.* He lives in Bozeman, Montana, with his wife and young son.

HAIKUS
BY Z.J. CZUPOR

Who wrote this mystery?
This novel virus that kills
The author be damned!

———

WHO believes China.
Who believes WHO and Fauci?
Who here knows the truth?

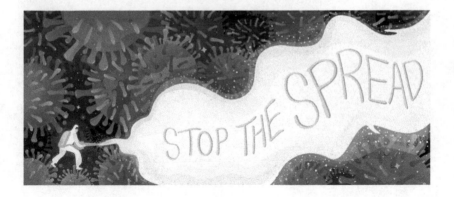

Experts know what's what
You can count on them for truth
...Unless they are wrong.

———

The crack of the bat
A sound missing from us now
Do we blame a bat?

PART II

COPING

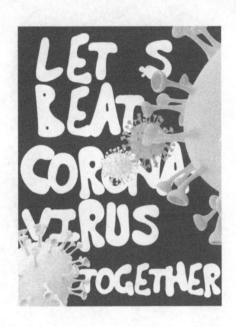

7

THE FIVE STAGES OF CORONANXIETY

BY SARAH M. CHEN

A CONVERSATION WITH—

- **S: Sarah**, anxious woman living in Los Angeles
- **D: Sarah's dad**, lives with his wife, Mian, in Taiwan
- **M: Sarah's mom** who lives near her

STAGE ONE: FEAR FOR MY DAD

February 17, 2020

S: Dad! Someone in Taichung has died of the virus!

D: [groan]

S: Hello? Dad? [pause] It's already nine a.m. in Taiwan. You're not up yet?

D: [yawn]

S: Aren't you worried? Someone from your town has died of the virus!

D: I know. [clears throat] It was a taxi driver with pre-existing conditions.

S: Are you wearing a mask? Are you staying inside? You're not going to restaurants, are you?

D: [sigh]

S: Don't tell me you're still swimming in the public pool.

D: [pause] I need my exercise.

S: STOP SWIMMING IN THE PUBLIC POOL!

D: They take our temperature first.

S: I don't care. Pools are petri dishes. I'm telling you right now not to swim! [pause] Dad? [pause] Hello?

STAGE TWO: FEAR FOR MYSELF

February 21, 2020

S: Are you and Mian still coming to L.A. and staying with me?

D: Yes.

S: [pause] What if you have the virus and pass it on to me?

D: I feel fine. I don't have the virus.

S: [silence]

D: Don't worry. Ever since SARS in 2003, Taiwan has been prepared for something like this. They take our temperature everywhere we go. They're rationing masks.

S: [silence]

D: I stopped swimming.

S: [sigh] Thank you. [pause] I'll check in with you later.

FEBRUARY 22, 2020

S: Mom?

M: Hi, honey.

S: You still want me to bring Dad and Mian over for lunch when they're in town?

M: Sure.

S: Really? You're not worried at all?

M: About what?

S: [silence]

. . .

STAGE THREE: ANGER

February 23, 2020

S: Okay. What dates are you staying with me?

D: Mian and I will be flying to Seattle for a wedding on March 6. Then we'll stay with you in L.A. on the way back to Taiwan which will be—.

S: WAIT, WHAT?

D: We will be flying to Seattle—

S: Are you trying to get the coronavirus?

D: It's all arranged already.

S: Cancel it.

D: Mian's brother is there now. If he says it's not safe, we'll cancel.

S: What's he going to say? I see the virus but we're steering clear of it?

D: If the wedding is called off, we won't go.

S: The bride is not going to call off her own wedding. [pause] Who is this selfish bitch who is having a wedding in the hot zone in the middle of a pandemic?

D: Your stepmother's only niece.

S: Well, I hope it rains on her wedding day!

MARCH 6, 2020

S: How are you feeling? Are you okay?

D: We went to Pike Place Market today.

S: [long silence]

D: Hello?

S: Was it crowded?

D: Yes, there were a lot of people around.

S: [silence]

D: We went to the first Starbucks. There was a long line.

S: Did you stand in it?

D: We did at first. But there were too many people so we gave up.

S: Were people standing far apart from each other?

D: No.

34

S: Dad, you need to stay in your hotel room and not come out. Stop sightseeing right this second.

D: Don't be silly.

S: Stop being so stubborn! You're taking a huge risk by being there. You're risking your life, Mom's life, and mine!

STAGE FOUR: GUILT

D: Then I won't stay with you when we arrive in L.A. And we won't visit your mother.

S: [silence]

D: Okay? I think it's best for everyone.

S: Stop it. You're staying with me, goddammit.

D: Okay.

STAGE FIVE: ACCEPTANCE

March 11, 2020

S: How was your flight back to Taiwan? Did you wipe everything down? How are you feeling? Are you okay?

D: Yes.

S: It was great having you here, Dad. I'm sorry if I was a little anxious.

D: That's okay.

S: And I'm sorry for wiping everything you and Mian touched with Clorox wipes.

D: That's okay. I understand.

S: [sigh] Thank you.

D: I enjoyed our time together.

S: Me too. [pause] I'm glad you're back safe in Taiwan. I'll call you tomorrow. See how you're feeling.

D: Please do.

S: I love you, Dad.

D: Love you back.

· · ·

IN HINDSIGHT, I needn't have worried so much about my dad. Taiwan has been applauded worldwide for its swift response to COVID-19. As of June 1, Taiwan has had only 443 cases and seven deaths. When Taiwan confirmed its first case in January 2020, President Tsai Ing-wen immediately sprang into action, putting restrictions on travel and ensuring the availability of medical supplies and personal protective equipment for the island. Temperatures continue to be monitored at airports, all High Speed Rail stations, schools, and restaurants. Masks are rationed to two per person per week through their universal health care system.

My dad and I continue to talk every night on the phone. What started as a check-in on each other's health has transformed into an evening ritual that I cherish. Our conversations serve as a gentle reminder that despite my coronanxiety, everything turned out okay. I still worry about him but instead of allowing my anxiety to take over, I channel that energy into gratitude for what I do have: my family, my health, and a growing hope for our future.

SARAH M. CHEN has published numerous short stories and a children's book. Her noir novella *Cleaning Up Finn* was an Anthony finalist and IPPY Award winner. She is the co-editor, along with E.A. Aymar, of *The Swamp Killers* and *The Night of the Flood*. She's written for the *Los Angeles Review of Books, Intrepid Times, Hapa Mag,* and *P.S. I Love You*.

8

BE CAREFUL WHAT YOU WISH FOR
BY JACQUI BROWN

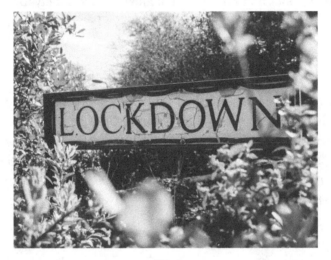

courtesy Matt Seymour

I CAN'T REMEMBER how many times over the last fifteen years I've wished that my life could stay within the small French village we call home. Whether it was yet another early morning school run I couldn't face, a wild and windy airport run I could have done without, or just the fact that being here makes me feel safe and happy, there have been many times I've dreaded getting in the car and driving away. Well, as from midday today, this village will be my life.

In an attempt to restrict the spread of the pandemic virus Covid-19, President Macron has closed down France. Borders have been shut, all non-essential shops and business have been closed, all social gatherings are forbidden and leaving the house has to be for a justified reason.

I can only feel relief at the happy coincidence that my husband Adrian and our 19-year-old son Ed both came home last Thursday, just hours before President Macron's first address to the nation. It was at this point we realized that neither of them would be leaving me, or the village, for quite some time as universities were to be closed, and Adrian's work as a freelance trainer; travelling Europe and working from a different office each week, is no longer tenable with the current situation. As someone who is so often home alone things feel far less scary knowing we are all here together and not in three different locations, as is our norm.

FEELING Positive

Our first full day of lockdown and we awoke to a perfect day. The sun was burning through the mist and by the time we took our breakfast outside, the sky was blue, and the birds were singing. Adrian being far more observant than I am noticed what was missing: the aircraft. Our sky is usually crisscrossed with plane trails, but this morning it was clear and quiet. I'm sure we will see an improvement in air quality in the coming weeks and that has to be a positive thing. Maybe this virus was the something dramatic needed by the planet to stop us in our tracks and save our futures?

I am still bubbling with the excitement you get at the beginning of a holiday. It is not often I get both Ed and Adrian home together for more than a long weekend and I'm going to enjoy every moment of this enforced family time. We are lucky to have a house that feels much too large when it's just me rattling around but offers each of us space to do our own thing when we need it.

A new routine

It might only be day three, but I have noticed our lives have slipped into a new routine already. Adrian and I are up around eight o'clock. We've been lucky enough to have breakfast in the garden every day and the house and village are peaceful enough for Adrian to work and me to write. By the time we stop for a late morning coffee, Ed is opening his shutters and his breakfast is usually a similar time to our lunch. The afternoon and early evening are family time; working outdoors, eating dinner together and relaxing in front of the television. When Adrian and I head off to bed, Ed takes over the lounge and the TV and goes to bed at some point that doesn't exist in our 24-hour clock. I know teenagers can have a reputation for being lazy, but you won't hear me complaining.

For Ed, life has changed dramatically. At 19 and with the independence of a city center studio apartment with his girlfriend, the shock to be stuck back in a village in the middle of nowhere with just his parents must be hell on earth. However, he is a star and taking it all in his stride. He is not angry, sulky or any of the emotions I know would have been bursting out of me if I had been put in a similar position at his age. He is calm, chatty and helpful. By having our slightly staggered days, I think we stand a much better chance of getting through this without falling out.

CHANGE OF FOCUS

My current coping mechanism seems to involve the need to be as organized and in control at home as possible. In fact, this need has given me more drive and motivation than usual, almost as if lockdown has unlocked parts of my head that I have been struggling with for a while. Every task I achieve from clearing out the freezers, to ensuring there is always a homemade cake in the tin, to sorting out areas of house and garden that have festered for too long: all help to improve my mood. This increased activity is balanced by yoga and home cooked meals, which keep me feeling calm, grounded and sleeping well at night. We are all different. For Adrian, hard exercise is what he needs and for Ed it is his music.

In some bizarre way I think I needed this massive change of focus. Something big and beyond my control, forcing a rethink and taking the attention away from the doom and gloom of Brexit, that as a British family in France has hung over us for almost four years. This is bigger than Brexit and has the magnitude to create more harm and damage to our lives, but this time we are all in it together. This is an invisible war. We can't see the enemy approach; we can only try to protect ourselves and those around us to the best of our ability and do whatever is necessary to cope. If we are targeted, we just have to hope that we have the strength to recover.

––––––

JACQUI BROWN IS a blogger at http://www.frenchvillagediaries.com. A British expat, she has been living in southwest France with her husband Adrian and son Ed since August 2004.

9

SWEET PAIN

BY NAOMI HIRAHARA

DURING A PANDEMIC and several days before protests over another unjust police killing of a black man, our dog, Tulo, was diagnosed with liver cancer. He's a pound puppy, adopted from the Pasadena Humane Society when he was already the estimated advanced age of eight. We've had him for almost seven years. I was hoping that more of his life would be spent with us than the great unknown of the first half of his life.

So how to hold all of this in the same hands? The grief over the impending physical demise and death of a canine companion, the boredom of sheltering in place with homemade culinary delights our only satisfying communal diversion and watching the visceral rage and chaos over our racist legacy on a computer screen. It's all surreal. The isolation is debilitating and in some ways, I can understand the unbridled actions of rioters, the desire to express anger and frustration—both warranted and self-serving—in a real, tangible way.

On social media, the reactions to both the pandemic and race-related protests have been extreme. Some say our systems in place must be literally burnt to the ground to make room for something new. On the other side, people have said reactions to COVID-19 have been overblown. Business must continue as usual so that we don't enter another Great Depression.

I agonize through all of this. I admit that I'm personally conflict-averse, choosing to embrace unconditional love, grace, and harmony. But I also fully understand that only espousing such positivity is to maintain the status quo. True change—whether it be to wear an uncomfortable mask for the well-being of other people or to insist on racial and economic justice to be reflected in our established institutions—is painful. Over Zoom, I meet with about ten Southern Californians of faith—black, white, Latino and Asians and mostly women —to discuss the book, Rethinking Incarceration by Dominique DuBois Gillard. The material is heavy and I feel my mind expanding. I don't have more answers but I need to keep poking at my calcified self to keep it soft and open.

Not knowing how long this season will last, we continue through these days of the pandemic in pain. I check on my 84-year-old mother, who is spending her days mostly in her backyard garden in South Pasadena, tending flowering plants that she grew from cuttings that she received from friends. From a six-foot distance, I watch my 10-year-old nephew do magic tricks with a coin on my brother's porch. And I walk the streets of my neighborhood with Tulo, enjoying the shade of the jacaranda and oak trees and the sweet but short-lived fragrance of jasmine.

———

NAOMI HIRAHARA IS the Edgar Award-winning author of two mystery series set in Southern California. Her Mas Arai series, which features a Hiroshima survivor and Altadena gardener, ended with the publication of *Hiroshima Boy* in 2018. Her Hawai'I mystery, *Iced in Paradise*, was released in September 2019. Her new historic standalone set in 1944 Chicago, *Clark and Division*, will be published by Soho Crime in May 2021. A former editor of The Rafu Shimpo newspaper, she has also published noir short stories, middle-grade fiction and nonfiction

history books. She was born in Pasadena and lives there today. www.-
naomihirahara.com

10

THIS WILL COST YOU

BY CRAIG LANCASTER

WE DROVE into Montana on April 4, 2020. Eighteen days later—after the moving truck had been emptied into our new (old) condo, after we had adhered to and emerged from the governor's order of a four-teen-day quarantine, after we had set up housekeeping and accli-mated our pets to their new routines, after we had learned to negotiate the delivery services and all the pandemic-inspired new aspects of an old place, after I'd been diagnosed with shingles for crying out loud—my wife's uncle died.

And that, if you can believe it (and even if you can't), was the moment that we discovered one of the cruel tolls of the coronavirus and the disease it unleashed, Covid-19.

My wife's dear Uncle Ronnie—my dear Uncle Ronnie, whose first words to me ever were "I feel like I know you"—died alone in a New York hospital of complications from surgery. Covid-19 didn't take him, not directly, but it robbed everyone who loved him. It's still robbing us.

It robbed his kids of a chance to say goodbye at his bedside. It robbed his family of a funeral, a memorial service, a gathering of everyone who knew and loved him so they could talk about what a wonderful coworker he was, what a lovely baby brother he was, what a dedicated father he was, what a gifted guitar player he was.

It robbed my wife of a chance to get on a plane and go home, to be in the mournful embrace of family as everyone tries to figure out how life can possibly go on without Ronnie.

The cost is too high. It's too much. No one should have to pay it.

And yet, even as I write the preceding three sentences, I know that our burden is comparatively light. We're alive, if not entirely living as we once thought of it, while we wait for something resembling normalcy to return. As I put down these words, the U.S. death toll has crossed 50,000, a number surely to rise. Only in the awful solitude of my imagination do I dare consider what it might be before these words find your eyes. I don't want to know. But I'm going to. If I live to see the final toll. If I'm lucky. The word lucky has never been so perverse.

If you'll forgive the coldly corporate nomenclature, Covid-19 has a cost structure, and the tolls seem random: Some pay with isolation. Some pay with inconvenience. Some pay with sickness followed by recovery. Many millions have paid with their jobs. Tens of thousands, so far, have paid with their lives in the U.S. Worldwide, it's hundreds of thousands more.

The only bitterly sure thing is that we're all paying with something.

We had no designs on moving during a pandemic. Our house in Maine—a lovely home in a lovely place that wasn't lovely enough to hold us from returning to Montana—went on the market in September 2019, when the world was in comparative bliss. It went under contract in mid-January, when the coronavirus was known but abstract, when the machinations of government that we would have silently expected to kick in and keep us safe were, in fact, doing nothing of the sort. As the grim reality came clear, we held our breath and waited and hoped for the closing, even as we knew what we'd be up against as we transported our lives across twelve states. On March 30, we began heading west.

The move was surreal. Empty turnpikes in New York and Pennsylvania and Ohio. We took heart. People were treating this seriously. I gassed up both cars—Elisa and the cat in one, me and my eighty-year-old father and two dogs in another—while wearing a mask and rubber gloves. I checked us into our hotel rooms in Buffalo and Chicago and Minneapolis and Bismarck. I ordered our food from Door Dash and made my own deliveries. We never felt safer than in the cars, with all that endless driving.

The move was maddening. The farther west we traveled, as the hotspots fell away, the more cavalier people seemed about the pandemic. In Janesville, Wisconsin, I walked into a store and turned around on my heel, the crowding of people without masks an unthinkable risk. In a rest area bathroom, I told an encroaching man to back the hell up. "I'm not sick," he said. "But what if I am?" I countered. In North Dakota, I was mocked for my mask. "Did it ever occur to you," I asked the man, "that I'm wearing this for your protection?" That shut him up.

They're all going to pay. I don't say that with a sense of vengeance. I just know that they are. We all are. The toll is inescapable. The only question is, at what rate will they be billed?

Finally, at last, the move was a relief. We're in Montana. We're in our place. We're healthy, shingles notwithstanding. We're taking precautions even as we continue to see others act in a way that suggests they're untouchable.

They're not.

It can be as simple and as punishing as this: You wake up one morning and you learn that your uncle is dead. Your mother, his big sister, is in the throes of pain two thousand miles away. In any other time, you could go to her, and to your other loved ones, and commune in your shared devastation.

This, however, is not that time.

Oh, you're going to pay.

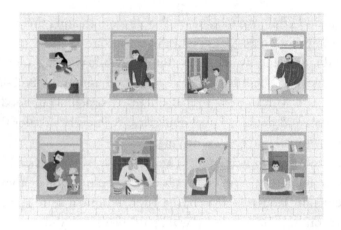

CRAIG LANCASTER WAS ONCE CALLED "one of the most important writers in Montana," and it wasn't even his mother who said it. (It was David Crisp, the founder and editor of the late, lamented Billings Outpost.) He's written eight published novels, notably the High Plains Book Award-winning *600 Hours of Edward,* as well as a collection of short stories. He's a staff editor at the sports journalism site The Athletic and also serves as the design director of and a frequent contributor to Montana Quarterly magazine.. He lives in Billings, Montana, with his wife, novelist Elisa Lorello. www.craig-lancaster.com

11

BEST LAID PLANS AND THE VIRUS: A CAUTIONARY TALE

BY WENDY HORNSBY

THE TIME HAD COME, no more delays. We were finally going back to France after several years of plans getting shuffled aside by one thing or another. After the holidays, we told family and friends we would visit, and before the spring break mobs arrive. Datebooks were compared, an itinerary was set. Northern France first, then southern Germany, a sweep through the Loire Valley, and finally a nice long stay in Paris in a hotel just steps away from the apartment my mystery series character, Maggie MacGowen, inherited from her mother. If the apartment, and Maggie, actually exist only in fiction, they are very real to me. I was truly looking forward to retracing her steps, revisiting favorite places, discovering new ones. And gathering material for another book or two.

Airline tickets bought and hotel reservations made, luggage pulled down from the shelf, passports up to date: we were set to go. Then, out of China, came news of a strange new virus with a science fiction worthy name, COVID-19. Someone ate under-cooked cobra? Or maybe a bat? It sounded exotic, and it was far, far away. But by the time we boarded our plane for Paris, the insidious virus had made its way into other parts of Asia via cruise ship passengers and trade, we were told, and had hit Italy with a vengeance. We weren't going anywhere near Italy's locked-down borders, so instead of turning around and going home, we blithely forged on.

For years we have quietly wiped down our area on an airplane with sanitary wipes before buckling up because we have seen what people do in those cramped little spaces, so of course we carried a supply. We are good about washing our hands and would do our best to keep them away from our faces as people were now being told. Careful people thus prepared, what could touch us? We were healthy, protected, bulletproof, and in a profound state of denial.

The first weeks of our trip were glorious, full of adventure and discovery and people we enjoy spending time with. For the most part, the virus kindly remained somewhere else, though every day we were made more aware of its spread. Then, suddenly, during the second week of March, the virus was global, a pandemic now. Everyone, everywhere was in peril if drastic and immediate action wasn't taken to stop its progress. Nations of Europe began shutting down schools and businesses, closing borders. The American response was slow, unclear, and seemed to shift from one hour to the next. Was no one allowed into the U.S.? Could citizens return? Might we be in Europe for an indefinite time?

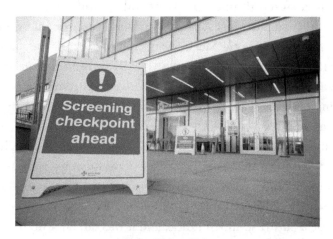

courtesy Graham Ruttan

Various friends offered their guest rooms if we got stuck. But not knowing how long the shutdowns might last, or what they might include, we decided to call our travel agent and ask her to cancel the rest of our trip. No Paris, no Germany, no lingering in gardens, castles, or museums anywhere, for now. We needed to go home.

During those chaotic early days, airline ticket agents were overwhelmed with calls as people scrambled to do exactly what we were trying to do—go home. After much effort, our agent managed to rebook our flights, but the earliest available was still five days away. During those five days, we felt as if we were running in the face of an avalanche as facility after facility that we relied on shut down. Our hotel in Strasbourg closed at noon the day we left. Restaurants across France had closed the night before.

Never were we in danger of going hungry or having to sleep in our rental car. The lurking danger was the virus, and the most dangerous place to be, it seemed to us, was anywhere near an international airport crammed with anxious people. We hoped that over the next five days, while we sheltered somewhere, the situation would settle and our passage out wouldn't be as fraught as the airport scenes we watched on televised news.

The owner of the isolated chateau in the Loire Valley where we had rooms booked for the following weekend, graciously allowed us to come and stay. Markets and bakeries were open so no one starved. Far from it. The afternoon before the first of the six cancelled or rescheduled flights in our future was set to depart, we headed to an airport adjacent to the hotel. Before dawn the next morning, we arrived at Charles deGaulle to learn that hours before, unclear—the airline's words—on the meaning of the American president's new restriction on incoming passengers from Europe, all flights to the U.S. were canceled. Gate agents rebooked us for the following morning with the caveat that they did not know if that flight would also be canceled. It was. Rebooked again, this time connecting through Munich, we were told to remain optimistic that if the flight left Paris the connecting flight would leave Munich, and if it did cross the Atlantic to be prepared to be redirected to any of the five American airports accepting European flights, and to understand that if we did reach the U.S. we could be locked into quarantine who knows where for a couple of weeks.

We girded our loins, gathered our luggage yet again, and headed into the mass of anxious humanity at the airport. Long lines, a crush of people stuck in close contact. This time, the plane actually took off. As did the next, and the next, even if not on schedule. And thirty hours later, not the usual ten, we were back where we began all those weeks before.

Regrets? None. Disappointment the trip was cut short? No. What we had seen and done while we were in France was magic enough for now. We'll go back, when it's safe. In the meantime, I have collected enough material for a book or two. Or three.

———

AN NPR INTERVIEWER APTLY DESCRIBED Edgar-Award winning author Wendy Hornsby as "a genteel college professor by day, and by night a purveyor of murder most foul." Now Professor of History Emeritus, she has abandoned all pretense of gentility in order to purvey stories of foul murder full time. She is the author of fifteen books and many short stories. *A Bouquet of Rue*, (Perseverance Press, April 2019), her most recent Maggie MacGowen mystery, is available now, and her story, "Ten Years, Two Days, and Six Hours," can be found in *Deadly Anniversaries* (Hanover Square Press, April 2020). www.wendy-hornsby.com

ODE TO THE CITY

BY WENDY SALINGER

What's a city?

I forget.
My stanzas are bare as winter now,
though I still feel the presence of the crowd
sometimes, like a hand at my shoulder.

In towns and suburbs I was lonely.
I wanted to be lost.
Those first weeks after I came
I walked for hours without a destination,

letting the multitudes stream past
like a soothing wind In my face.
I wanted to feel the structure
as it moved around me

and myself inside it
like an alto inside four-part harmony,

a pinball jostled between the alleys
until I found my place.

I wanted to hear every story.
On buses and park benches
people translated furiously for me
into French, into Spanish, into Garifuna.

Museums magnified me.
I breathed easier in those rooms
where the elusive present lingered
In the echoes of the past.

I wanted life to tower over me, to stand on corners
where buildings with the skins of mirrors
ricocheted and multiplied off each other
so I could be everywhere at once.

What's a city?

Twice each year the sun tries to grasp It,
from low on the horizon, extending its arms,
each spoke an ancient, toppled column
lying west to east, Illuminating all the frames.

And now we too, at sunset, gather to remember
at every level—from balcony
to mezzanine to orchestra pit,
our windows thrown open

like those on an Advent calendar
in the depths on December,
banging our earthly utensils till we become
like sounding brass and tinkling cymbal,

shouting our praise for this thing that's our own creation
and for the deeds of the men and women
as they set out to care for it
beneath unfathomable skies.

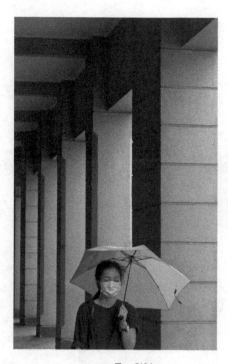

courtesy Tam Wei

AFTER WE'RE GONE

BY WENDY SALINGER

After we're gone
The narrator
Will keep telling the story.

Who will it be?
Who will pick up the thread
And redraw the sun

And the moon
And the stars
And the empty horizon?

March, 2020

Wendy Salinger's memoir *Listen* (Bloomsbury, 2006), was nominated for The Krause Essay Prize. Her book of poetry *Folly River*

(Dutton, 1980), was the winner of the first Open Competition of The National Poetry Series. She lives in New York City where she directs The Walker Literature Project at the 92nd Street Y.

PART III

STORIES FROM AROUND THE GLOBE

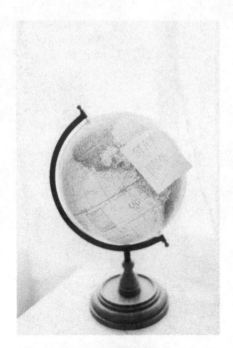

courtesy Bruno Cervera

12

THE LOFT

BY GEORGE ARION - ROMANIA

Translated from Romanian by Mihnea Arion

I'M GOING NUTS!

For two months now I've been living as if under house arrest, for fear of the new Coronavirus, strictly observing the rules imposed by the authorities.

"STAY HOME!" has been this year's motto – you do otherwise, you show them the money. Lots of it.

I only go out between 11AM and 1PM, when people over sixty-five are allowed to purchase the groceries in shops close to their home.

Of course, every time I go out, I am required to carry a pass on me which specifies why I'm going out. I also wear a mask and gloves to protect myself from the villainous virus whenever I put my hands on things which others have touched.

At the cashier, I stand two meters away from the guy in front and I make sure the guy behind stands two meters away from me.

Things are still alright, shelves full, just like normal times. I don't even dare imagine the potential chaos with nothing to put on the table.

But I've had it with the contradictory news on TV, the fights between politicians more concerned with inflating their own popularity than finding solutions to the crisis, the constant reruns on networks which can't afford to buy new movies.

I'm bored to death.

Nobody's allowed to come and visit and I'm not in the mood to meet some potentially contaminated individual anyway. I've even stopped going to my shrink so, naturally, I've blasted through my stockpile of prescription pills.

I'm all alone.

My head hurts and I've started seeing and hearing things, shadows creeping in corners, strange voices whispering.

The panic attacks have become more frequent as well.

The isolation I'm forced to endure breeds monsters.

I've become a creature unable to recognize its own home anymore.

Recently, however, I've found myself a pastime that should do away with the monotony of isolation.

I've started spying on a woman.

Whoa, no dirty thoughts here! I'm just studying another human being.

She lives in a loft in the apartment building opposite mine. Her window's always open, even at night, with a chill wind blowing. I watch her conscientiously, so I know when she leaves the house and comes back, when she goes to sleep or wakes up in the morning – but I've never seen her face. Indeed, from the lookout where I watch over the bustling street or contemplate what sort of life pigeons lead on rooftops I can only see her legs, below the knees. Through the narrow window of her loft I also glimpse a bed, an armchair where she sometimes rests with her legs crossed, a coffee table and a carpet.

The woman leads a secluded life. I've never seen anyone else in her loft.

How is she holding up, I wonder?

Every so often, tunes by Bach, Beethoven and others flow outside from her window. She listens to them on an old phonograph with the volume cranked up.

I must admit, I find her intriguing. So, for some time now, whenever I see her put on her shoes – she wears slippers indoors, I think they must be very comfy – I lean outside way over the windowsill to see her walk out.

But every time I look there's either nobody coming out, or, if a woman does come out, her legs aren't the ones I like to contemplate – marvelous, unmistakable, slim ankles, muscles that seem to effortlessly move and slice through the air.

I then tell myself she must've changed her mind and decided she doesn't want to go out anymore. I glance at the room across the street – there's nobody there. I stalk the entrance again – there's no woman there to catch my eye. And yet, in the evening, I see light through her window but have no idea when she's come back.

My headaches are getting worse. My temples are throbbing like mad. My vision is often clouded. I have vertigo and one morning I almost slip in the bathroom. I manage to regain my balance, but I still end up with a nice bruise.

I can't stand it anymore!

Finally, the quarantine is over. Now I can pay her a visit and meet her. I'm going to ring her bell, ready to fire a random excuse.

Of course, I could have predicted that the elevator would be out of order today, but it's not the end of the world to climb up to the fifth floor. However, the climb triggers my vertigo. I lean on a wall for a few moments to catch my breath.

I'm at her door. I hesitate. I want to ring the bell, but the door's ajar. I push it and step in a small hallway. A wave of fever washes over me. I struggle to keep my increasing anxiety under control.

I look around.

On a coat rack I see neatly arranged clothes. I take a few steps on a tiny carpet and end up in front of another door. This one's ajar as well. I push it firmly.

My heart's about to burst.

My nerves are strained to the limit.

I'm about to faint.

For a second, I close my eyes to compose myself.

When I open them again I freeze: inside the room there's a pair of legs walking around. Long, lovely, with fine ankles – but no body.

———

GEORGE ARION IS a Romanian journalist famous for his interviews and also an author who writes multiple literary genres - poetry, prose, drama and essays. He is the author of movie and TV scripts, as well as of an opera libretto. He has been thrice awarded with The Romanian Writers' Union prize and also with the Romanian Writers' Association prize. His novels have been translated into English, French, Macedonian and Russian. The translator of this story, Mihnea Arion, is his son.

13

COUNTRY LIFE IN THE TIME OF CORONAVIRUS

BY EOGHAN EGAN - IRELAND

'Is Mother Nature taking revenge on us or is she planning a rebirth?' Mickey Brennan's elbow rested on the top bar of the five-metre long field gate and he eyed his neighbour, Jim Kelly, who was leaning against the other end.

Jim lifted his cap, scratched his head, swatted at a red-tailed bumblebee and turned to salute a passing car. 'People tell me life's gonna return to normal within a few weeks,' he said, settling the cap back in place. 'But I think it'll take months, even years.'

'Aye. Diya know what a man told me yesterday?'

'What?'

'He said farmers will hafta become digital entrepreneurs in order to survive.'

'Digital entrepreneurs?' Jim blinked and squinted at the field of sheep. 'How'll that work?'

'Well,' Mickey stooped, picked up a blade of grass, examined it, and straightened. 'He reckons we won't be let into marts on account of social distancing, an' dealers won't come to our yards, so we'll have to sell stock online by taking photos of the animals, type out a description, an' create an online... advertisement, like the way those fellas selling cars do it.'

'An' how'll we get paid?'

'Sure, that's all done online too.' Mickey chewed on the grass blade. 'Any dealing will be done by phone, an' money'll be in your bank account before the buyer collects his stock from some state approved disinfected zone. Cash is dead. Digital entrepreneurs will be the new kings.'

'Huh. An' I bet it won't be long before some boyo with a college degree who doesn't know a heifer from a bullock will make himself a middleman and look for a cut,' Jim added. 'Speaking of degrees, how's your daughter, the doctor, getting on?'

'Up to her eyes with this virus.'

'Can't she take sick leave, or holidays?' Jim said. 'If it was me, I'd—'

'Nah. Leave's suspended. All hands on deck. Least she can head home after working her shift, not like some patients. Yesterday she had to tell a forty year-old man's family that he'd been confirmed positive, and because of some heart problem, he wouldn't survive. An hour later she told an eighty year-old woman she'd be going home. This virus...' Mickey shook his head. '...it's a killer if you've other health issues. People need to start taking responsibility for their actions. It mightn't affect you or me too bad, but pass it on to an older person, an' next stop's the funeral parlour. This thing of townies heading off to their holidays homes...' Mickey shook his head again.

'So long as she's safe,' Jim said.

'Aye. She is, thank God. It's the not being able to treat her Covid-19 patients with a vaccine that's gettin' to her, though. All she can do is keep them comfortable and see if bodies heal themselves... or don't. That's what it boils down to.' Mickey gazed at the sheep. 'Coronavirus takes no prisoners.'

'How's your uncle managing?' Jim turned to face Mickey.

'Not a bother. Phoned him last night, asked him if he needed anything. He said, "I'm eating well, sleeping well and keeping busy." 'Busy doing what?' says I. "Busy doing nothing," he said.' Mickey cackled like an angry goose. He shaded his eyes, squinted into the distance and gestured towards a dot half-way up the distant mountain. 'See? There's smoke rising from his chimney. We're lucky out here with lots of space and fresh air.'

Mickey shifted another centimetre away from Jim. 'Us country folk are used to dealing with everything from parasites to pandemics, but this one's a whole different ball game.' Mickey spat out the well-chewed grass blade. 'I'd better be getting back or the missus will have an all-points bulletin out for me. She's organising a few home grown vegetable food parcels for me to deliver around the neighbourhood. An' she's got one of those new-fangled temperature scanners. Spent yesterday waving it around like a handgun. Even the dog got its temperature taken fifty times. You're lucky to have young 'un's in your house. They take some of the pressure off you.'

'Lucky? Me?' Jim grimaced. 'Ya must be joking. They say it takes a village to rear a child, well, let me tell you, it takes a bloody good-sized distillery to home-school them. Especially with our hit 'n' miss broadband signal. Teaching is... complicated. I'll never begrudge Mary Kelly her long summer holidays again.'

'Aye. 'Wasn't it shocking I couldn't even sympathise with Mary on her father's—'

'Ah, poor Bob. God rest his soul. He went fast in the end. I knew the man all my life. He taught me how to—'

'I know he did. Desperate that I'd to watch a friend's funeral mass on a video stream. Even his ninety year-old mother wasn't allowed near the church, or be at his graveside for the burial. That's tough.'

Jim nodded. 'Tis.'

'He liked his pint, did Bob.' Mickey smacked his lips. 'I'm tellin' you now, I'll never refuse an opportunity to go to the pub again. I'm gasping for a real pint of Guinness with a good thick creamy head. Aww man, I can taste it.'

'We'll have to wait.' Jim pushed away from the gate and turned left. 'See you tomorrow?'

'Aye. If the missus doesn't shoot me with her temperature gauge.' Mickey turned right.

'Hey,' Jim called his friend.

Mickey turned.

'Maybe it's my imagination', Jim said, 'but last night, I was looking at the stars and they seemed clearer. To answer your question, I don't think Mother Nature's either taking revenge on us or planning a rebirth. I think she's healing herself.'

———

A NATIVE OF Co. Roscommon, Ireland, Eoghan wrote his first story aged nine. A graduate of Maynooth University's Creative Writing Curriculum, Eoghan divides his time between Roscommon, Dublin, and Southern Italy. The first in his trilogy of crime fiction novels, *Hiding in Plain Sight*, was released in January 2020. https://eoghanegan.com/

14

LIFE LINES

BY ADRIANA LICIO - ITALY

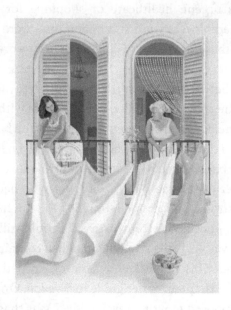

GIÒ BRANDO WOKE up as a sparkling ray of sunlight hit her bed. She stretched her arms, yawned, and for an instant she felt full of life, almost to the point of euphoria. She didn't even bother to look for her slippers before her feet were walking onto the small terrace of her attic flat.

It was the first truly pleasant day after an unusually long winter in southern Italy. The Mediterranean was glittering under the bright sunshine, the rocky mountains that embraced Giò's picturesque hometown of Maratea appearing to be clothed in the lushest green. Even the conic shape of Mount Bulgheria, on the other side of the Policastro Gulf, was clearly visible, blue and imposing in the distance.

Her eyes focused on details closer to home, the carpet of red roofs stretching out under her terrace, her mind already planning a good, long hike, or maybe she'd take a kayak out on the sea for the first time this season. Then the breath of the cool breeze, carrying the perfume of pine trees and sea, brought her back to the present. It was the end of March 2020, the third week of lockdown. Coronavirus was holding the world hostage. She couldn't go out, unless her reason for leaving her home was urgent: healthcare or shopping for food. The few people whose employers were still operational were allowed out to work, too, but that didn't affect Giò. She mainly worked from home anyway.

Reality hit her like a slap in the face. She left the balcony door open, despite the cool air, and filled her Moka pot with ground coffee. No chance to breakfast on a cornetto today – all the bars were closed. But, she still had the milk frother her sister had given to her when she had first come back from the UK to live in Maratea after the disastrous end of her engagement to a Londoner who had turned out to be... well, disastrous. She grinned, brandishing the metallic tool like a weapon. A cappuccino was one luxury she could still indulge in.

She laid her table, just a napkin and a dish containing a few rosemary and lavender biscuits baked by Granny, opened her laptop and read through the chapters of her guide to Sweden. On lockdown, and she was still supposed to write travel guides? Was that a blessing or a curse? She wasn't sure.

Concentration was hard to come by. Was her job going to survive in the new world that would emerge from the crisis? Or would it be wiped out? Would travel turn into a luxury for the privileged few? What was waiting for her at the end of the tunnel?

In the meantime, she wasn't even free to go and write at Leonardo's bar in Maratea's main square. She couldn't enjoy a coffee with her friends, nor indulge in late night chats with Paolo, the carabiniere with whom she had shared a few investigations and misadventures.

Birds were chirping outside, indifferent to the crisis, but it was one particular chirp that captured Giò's attention. It came not from the sky, nor from the trees, but from below, and it was too familiar to be ignored. Closing her laptop in exasperation, Giò returned to her terrace.

Two stories below, she could see Granny leaning from the back of her flat, hanging the laundry on the lines that stretched between her building and the one opposite, a few meters away. She and Anna, her neighbor, were chatting merrily from their windows, discussing food preparation and enquiring after family members. Then, by using one of the empty lines as a pulley system, Granny sent a small wicker basket over to Anna, and the woman gratefully pulled out the jar it contained.

"THANK YOU SO MUCH, Rosa, we simply love your orange marmalade. I will use it for our crêpes today. How are Agnese and the children?"

"She's had to close her shop, so she's quite worried. The times ahead are not going to be easy, but I was born just before the war and I keep telling her we've come through far worse. We still have food to eat. The doctors and nurses, as tired as they might be, are still there for us."

"I see, poor Agnese. It's the same for us – my husband is worried he won't have a job at the Pellicano Hotel this season..."

"I'm sure the authorities will do something to help tourism. It won't be a busy season, but we need to be resilient. By the way, how's Mrs. Mandarino? The poor woman is all by herself..."

"As a matter of fact, I'm here." A quavery voice sounded from a flat a few floors above Anna's. "Sorry if I was eavesdropping, but your voices were keeping me company."

"I was just thinking of you. I've prepared some lasagne for the family, but I have a portion set aside for you. Would you mind, Anna?" asked Granny, placing a dish in the wicker basket that Anna had sent back.

"Not at all," Anna said, pulling the basket over on the laundry line once more. Extracting the dish from Granny's basket, she put it into a second one that Mrs. Mandarino had lowered with a rope from her third-floor window.

"Thank you so much," the elderly lady said.

"If you want, we can eat together," Granny suggested. "At half past one, if that's not too late. I can sit here at the window."

"Sounds good to me, and the sun will be shining on our flats at that time. It will keep us warm."

As the three women chattered on, more baskets of goodies travelling along the laundry lines, Giò was reminded of a story Granny used to tell her when she was a child.

The people of Naples were misbehaving, lying, cheating and committing all sorts of foul crimes, so God decided to punish them with torrential rainfall that would leave none of them alive.

"Please, Lord," an angel asked, "if You're determined to proceed, may I ask You in Your wisdom to save one little girl? She's always done her duty and said her prayers."

God consented and sent the angel to save the little girl. But when he picked her house up to bring it to safety, the building next door came along too. Then another followed, and another. As the angel rose into the sky, it looked as though the whole city would be saved, as each house was linked to many others by simple laundry lines...

"Love runs along those lines," Granny would conclude.

A voice shrilled from beneath her. "Giò, come out and lower your basket. I've got some lasagne for you."

Giò did as she was asked. She'd be fine. In Maratea, there would always be a line of love running into her life.

———

ITALIAN AUTHOR ADRIANA LICIO spent 6 years in her beloved Scotland, and has never recovered. She lives somewhere in the Apennine mountains in southern Italy and whenever she can, rushes to Maratea, the seaside setting of her Italian Village Mystery series, featuring travel writer Giò Brando. When not under lockdown, she also runs her family perfumery shop. https://adrianalicio.com

15

THE DURATION

BY PIET TIEGELER - SPAIN

SHE HAD CONTRACTED the disease and he never saw her again. No goodbyes, no last words, immediate dispatch from the IC-unit to the undertaker.

Friday 3/13. They were lunching at their favorite restaurant when, all of a sudden, the world changed. The restaurant closed the same evening for an indeterminate time. Spain, like the rest of the world, went into lockdown.

Emile was a widower and Louise was a divorcée. They had met during a walking tour in the foothills of the Sierra, became friends and were soon considered a couple. Three months ago, Louise had given up the rented apartment in which she hibernated at the Costa, and came to stay in Emile's large villa.

Louise was a retired math teacher, proud of her steel-grey hair and her no-nonsense wardrobe. Emile was an elderly gentleman with romantic ideas. Louise told him to keep his feet on the ground, but one night when they were witnessing spectacular sundown on the terrace, she confessed to being happy.

All non-essential displacement was prohibited, the Guardia Civil controlled even supermarket tickets to prove that the groceries in the trunk of your car were bought in the last two hours. The highways were empty, the streets of the cities were eerily quiet. Housemaids stayed home and gardeners didn't show up. It became impossible to find a plumber or an electrician. Spain got the highest casualty rate of the Covid-19 pandemic and Louise decided to take the flight that offered Belgian citizens and residents the last chance to return home.

Emile was in doubt. He was a Belgian national, but he'd resided in Spain for more than twenty years. Louise told him that he was welcome to stay with her, but added that her apartment was tiny. Emile decided to stay where he was. He had four cats and a pond with goldfish and Louise promised to stay away only for the duration. She would use the opportunity to do all the paperwork for emigration to Spain and hurry back after the lockdown was lifted.

He drove her to the airport and they stayed in contact via Skype.

On April 10 Louise was not online at midday, their usual hour of contact. At 5 p.m. Emile received an SMS from her: 'have a fever, will have it checked. Love.'

Nothing after that.

Emile spent hours on the telephone, contacting hospitals but was not able to find a trace from Louise Janssens, the woman he loved and who had the most common surname in Belgium. Besides, was he her next of kin, or even a relative?

One by one Emile contacted the members of the walking club of their first encounter. He obtained the name of Louise's ex and got him on the telephone on April 27.

'Louise is dead,' said the man after Emile had haltingly explained who he was. There was an amount of sorrow in his voice, but also a trace of relief. Emile wondered if the man had paid alimony.

Money had not been an issue in Emile's relationship with Louise. Sometimes he paid, sometimes she did. The financing of their togetherness was of little concern.

'My wife was cremated,' said Louise's ex, 'and her ashes were scattered at the municipal burying ground. It had to be done immediately; infected corpses stay contagious.'

'Your wife? I thought...'

'We were separated, not divorced yet. I... ah.. am sorry for your loss.'

They said politely goodbye and Emile walked out on the terrace.

The sundown was as spectacular as ever and Emile decided not to move from here for the duration. The duration of his twilight years.

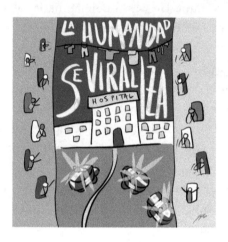

PIET TEIGELER MA was born in 1936 in Antwerp, Belgium. After retiring from journalism, he published 17 mystery novels in Dutch. Four were nominated for the Hercule Poirot Prize which he won in 2000 for 'The Black Death'. He was president worldwide of AIEP-IACW from 2003 until 2007 and has lived in Spain since 1998.

16

BREAK HIS BONE
BY MERRILEE ROBSON - CANADA

I DON'T KNOW that it was him.

But I still think he deserves to be punished.

I mean, it was Karl that went down to that demonstration. I saw him on the news with all those people, shouting about the right to work. Not that Karl was working before the lockdown. He had that insurance settlement and kept saying he was in too much pain to go back to work.

But that didn't stop him from marching around with a Confederate flag trailing behind him.

I didn't understand that. We're a northern state. And Karl was born here.

"C'mon, Rina," Karl said when I reminded him that Pete and I were working. "Other people want to work too. Don't you want to get your hair and nails done, go shopping? Go out to a restaurant?"

"People are supposed to stay home unless they have to go out," I told him. "To prevent the spread of the virus. To not be a burden on the health care system. To protect essential workers like me and Pete."

If we weren't at work at the grocery store, Pete and I stayed home. I thought Pete would be okay. He worked at night, stocking shelves when the store was closed. I was the one at the cash desk, dealing with customers all day.

That scared me.

I mean people need groceries; I get it. But Karl didn't need to be parading around with his buddies, no mask, no social distancing, no washing his hands when he got home.

And he could have left us alone.

"Come on over for a beer," he'd call when Pete got home from work.

And Pete, who never wanted to hurt anyone, would say no at first, saying he was tired.

"You need to unwind," Karl would say. "C'mon, just one beer."

And my Pete would say they should stay outside. Stay six feet apart. He'd try to wipe down the bottle that Karl handed him.

"Oh, you don't need to do that," Karl would say. "I'm not sick. This whole thing is just a hoax anyway. They're just trying to scare us."

"I didn't want to argue with him. The guy's just lonely," Pete would say.

And that's why I love my Pete. He didn't want to hurt anyone.

So I'd remind Pete to wash his hands. And when Karl borrowed our lawn mower, I'd make sure to wipe it down with disinfectant.

But when Pete started to cough, I knew it was Karl's fault.

I mean we never go anywhere. Just to work. And Pete works when no one else is around.

Where else could he have got it?

So when Pete had to go to the hospital and they started to talk about putting my Pete on a ventilator, I knew Karl needed to be stopped.

They talk in the Bible about an eye for an eye and a tooth for a tooth.

The pastor at a church I used to go to said it wasn't just from the Bible. Something about it being from a really old law called the Code of Hammurabi.

He told me it said something like, "If a man destroy the eye of another man, they shall destroy his eye. If one breaks a man's bone, they shall break his bone."

I like the bone breaking.

The pastor also said there were also rules in that code about not accusing someone if you can't prove it. But I don't know how they know what it says 'cause it was written in some language I don't think anyone speaks any more.

He said something about forgiveness too. I thought that was nice at the time.

Now, I took those tissues Pete had coughed blood into just before I took him to the hospital. I rubbed them on the handle of Karl's truck and his front door.

And those masks and disposable gloves that customers wear to the store and then just toss in the parking lot? I used those too, on the lawn chair he sits in when he drinks his beer. The rusted stair railing. On anything I thought he might touch.

After Pete got sick the store made me stay home. So it was easy. Whenever Karl went off to one of those rallies, to use the spare key he had given us to his house.

I'm not sick but I coughed on everything, over and over until my lungs hurt the way Pete said his hurt.

And I wiped the masks and gloves Pete had worn to work on the stuff in Karl's house. On the beer in his fridge, on the mugs in his cupboard, on the tap in his kitchen.

And on the handle of the lawnmower he always borrows from us.

They won't let me see Pete in intensive care.

So I've got time to look up that Code of Hammurabi.

I know it talks about breaking bones.

But what does it say about when a man dies? I need find that out.

———

A SERVANT TO TWO CATS, Merrilee Robson uses the time when the cats are sleeping to write mysteries. Fortunately, cats sleep a lot. Her first novel, *Murder is Uncooperative*, is set in a Vancouver housing co-op. Her short crime fiction has recently appeared in Ellery Queen Mystery Magazine, The People's Friend, Over My Dead Body, Mysteryrat's Maze podcast, Mystery Weekly, and other magazines and anthologies, including the upcoming Malice Domestic 15: Mystery Most Theatrical.. She lives in Vancouver, Canada. www.merrileerobson.ca.

GRAVEYARD CLOSED DUE TO COVID-19 LOCKDOWN *

BY PAUL JEFFCUTT

PRIESTS, morticians and mourners
　　barred until further notice.
　　Gatherings of two or more
　　ghouls will be dispersed.
　　Zombies without sanitizer
　　or hands are forbidden,
　　likewise the undead—
　　whether or not taking
　　essential exercise.
　　For their own safety,
　　the previously buried
　　are respectfully requested
　　to remain interred.

*GALLOWS HUMOR IS widespread amongst Medical and Emergency
Services personnel; it helps them to cope with the intense stress of
their working lives.

. . .

PAUL JEFFCUTT'S SECOND COLLECTION, 'The Skylark's Call,' is forth-coming from Dempsey & Windle; his first, 'Latch', was published by Lagan Press. Recently his poems have appeared in The Honest Ulsterman, Ink, Sweat & Tears, The Interpreter's House, Magma, Orbis, Oxford Poetry, Poetry Ireland Review, Poetry Salzburg Review and Vallum. He lives in Co Down, Northern Ireland. www.pauljeffcutt.net

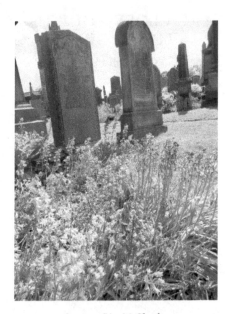

Courtesy Lise McClendon

SPENT *
PAUL JEFFCUTT

Candy, Bread, Microwave Meals,
Liquor, eCards, Sleeping Pills,
Pet Food, Chips, Video Streams,
Heroin, Wine, Computer Games,
Sausages, Butter, Toilet Rolls,
Cannabis, Cheese, Tylenol,
eBooks, Beer, Exercise Mats,
Vitamins, Cookies, Cold Cuts,
Ice Cream, Guns, Online Gambling,
Webcams, Eggs, Hair Coloring,
Chocolate, Bleach, Coffee,
Baked Beans, Tea, Pornography.

*the most popular products bought during lockdown

HAIKUS

BY Z.J. CZUPOR

Green grass. Flowers bloom.
I watch the spring from my room.
I long for your touch.

———

She's unemployed now
Spring blooms outside her window
Her smile disappears.

———

And the band plays on
Horns in LA, strings in Maine
They sound so Zoom-ie.

———

I pledge allegiance

One nation, under lockdown
For what do we stand?

PART IV

A WRITER'S MIND

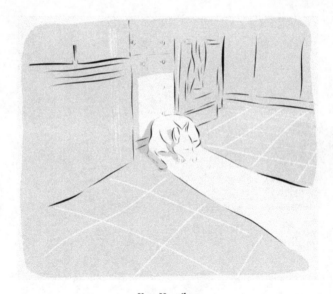

Kate Hourihan

17

THE QUARANTINE MURDERS
BY TATJANA KRUSE

IF POISON IS past its expiry date, is it more poisonous or is it no longer poisonous? I pondered.

It was a lazy late afternoon. I had just murdered a man and was sitting quietly on the balcony chair looking at the sunlit roofs in front of me, a coffee mug in my hand. I had no issues with life or the world. I was contemplating murder and mayhem, as usual. Which is absolutely fine as I am a mystery writer. And I only murdered the guy on paper.

That was the day before the Covid-19 lockdown in Germany.

When the good old days turned into Groundhog Day – others call it quarantine life – my muse wouldn't kiss me anymore.

The pandemic was an emotional roller coaster for me (as for everybody else, I guess.) Concern, poise, anxiety, aplomb, panic and every emotion in between.

I had always thought that no distractions whatsoever would be absolute paradise for me as a writer but as it turned out, my muse complied to the social distancing rules. This whole thing became a long distance flight of sorts where I was constantly snacking, binge-watching Netflix and drinking Gin and Tonic as early as too early.

. . .

IT IS a truth universally acknowledged that lockdown is going to prove one thing: most of us don't in fact have a novel in us "if only we had time to write." However, this – unfortunately – is true for professional writers as well in exceptional times like these.

For me, the unease, sometimes even the utter panic in the face of the pandemic and its economic consequences for us artists, had dried up the well of ideas.

Also, I didn't want to harm anyone anymore, not even fictitious characters who'd only get what they deserved. I wanted to spread goodwill and love to everyone. But my publisher didn't respond kindly to my inquiry whether they would print love haikus instead of book four of my detective series.

After about forty days of solitary confinement my muse suddenly returned. I have to thank my neighbors – the family of four from downstairs who constantly proved that sitcom family harmony is a lie. The ardent death metal fan from upstairs who seemed to have lost his headphones but was prone to open windows. The old lady with her two constantly barking dachshunds.

I. Was. Annoyed.

And in my annoyance suddenly I felt murderous again. Gone were love and goodwill. I yearned for blunt instruments, poisons, a SIG Sauer. Oh how I longed to slay them all. (Only on paper, of course. We mystery writers are all sweet, affable bunnies in real life because we act out our aggressions in our books.)

I fell in love with writing again. It became the driving force to get out of bed in the morning. There is no real point to life besides loving and laughing and living as best as we can, whatever the circumstances. Sometimes, you just have to grit your teeth and get on with it. Or as my granny used to say: "This, too, shall pass. Just put more sugar in your tea."

––––––

TATJANA KRUSE IS a mystery writer whose credits include the Sleuth Sisters Konny and Kriemhild, the needleworking Ex-Detective Siggi

Seifferheld and the Opera Singer/Private Eye Pauline Miller with her narcoleptic Boston Terrier Radames. In her former life, Tatjana worked as executive assistant, bookseller and literary translator. In her latest (and favorite) incarnation as a mystery novelist, she is a bestselling author and winner of several awards, including the Chandler Society's Marlowe award for Best German Short Story. She lives in the South of Germany. www.tatjanakruse.de

18

ISOLATION: A MINOR EPIPHANY
BY TIM CAHILL

I MAKE my living as a writer, and that means that when I work, I stay at home, see no one, and spend a bit of time tearing my hair out and kicking my desk and having intense literary discussions with my dog on our long daily walks. Self-isolation is nothing new to me. It's a way of life.

So, I have no problem with life in the pandemic-zone except, perhaps, for the fact that it has literally destroyed my profession. You see, I am a travel writer. Or I was. These days, people don't want to read about travel because they fear the very concept of leaving home. You might think this is overstated but I can tell you with great confidence that not one of my usual paying sources is clamoring for a Tim Cahill travel story.

I have been doing this work for just short of 50 years. My specialty was remote destinations and getting there generally involved backpacks and a lot of walking. I loved doing that stuff and had what I considered the best job in American journalism. But now, as a man in his mid-70s, I realize I'm in the crosshairs of the virus. There's a bunch of stuff I don't want to do anymore. I don't want to hang out overnight in a Nigerian airport or sit on a plane for 19 hours to get to Tasmania.

I thought, as I got older, various publications would switch me over to less strenuous assignments. A tour of the three-star Michelin restaurants of France. A luxury Mediterranean cruise on a private yacht. That sort of thing. I was looking forward to it.

But now, that's not going to happen. I mean, I'm stuck at home with no assignments, no deadlines, and nothing in the pipeline. Friends have urged me to write fiction and over the past few months I've given it a bit of a try. The results haven't been pretty. It turns out that my story about a guy on a tour of the three-star Michelin restaurants of France is a tasteless mélange of unappetizing morsels Googled up in a fruitless search for credibility. Fact is: I really don't care how they bruise the peppercorns.

When I try to write a thrilling mystery, I end up swimming in a soup of parody in which I make fun of the genre and of myself. Sex stories are out. I'll keep that to myself, thank you. Multi-generational novels spanning some great historical event ---Genghis Rising! --- might be okay but that means years of research and, as a history major, I'm over that. The truth is that, after a lifetime of writing non-fiction, of getting the details right, of having the facts checked, I'm incapable of writing about things I don't know for sure happened. This is not a trait common to major novelists.

And that is the one nearly important thing I've learned about myself in pandemic isolation: I suck at fiction.

––––––––

TIM CAHILL IS the author of nine books, one of which *National Geographic* named as one of the hundred best adventure travel books ever written. He lives in Montana.

19

EVERYONE DESERVES A CHANCE TO FOLLOW THEIR DREAMS

BY LISE MCCLENDON

THOSE WORDS WAFTED up from an actual dream as I slowly woke up. Like many writers my subconscious works best at these in-between times, the moments between waking and sleeping, that dreamy state where imagination lives. But what did that little piece of advice coming with an omniscient, slightly judgy voice— *aka* my mother— really mean?

The literal meaning is obvious, and something no one really argues against, right? Everyone DOES deserve a chance to follow their dreams. Having a dream about following a dream is pretty meta. I always enjoy being meta but— Why did this god-like voice tell me this that morning? What is my subconscious banging on about anyway?

The previous days had been normal, as normal as a pandemic can be. That is, fairly dull. My husband had left to visit his brother and scout out Montana for virus dangers, leaving me behind to feed the cat and carry on with my daily housekeeping and other inspiring chores. Let it be said I no longer resent the laundry, by the way. It gives structure to my day.

But I had seen very few people, and talked to even fewer. No one had FaceTimed me, and I had not reached out to do the same. (That was getting a little old. The first few 'happy hour' video chats were fun. Then you find yourself telling the same stories, over and over. Plus— makeup! Hair! Clean clothes!) My acquaintances in our newish second home community are not vast, as in a couple neighbors who must stay far away. The man who lives next door has been friendly and we've been getting to know him over the adjoining wall. Sometimes he stops and talks over the wall, *Home Improvement*-style. A few days before the dream he had just said hello and kept moving.

This was, of course, a nothing. But the isolation, without even a housemate to talk to, was obviously getting to me. Did I say something wrong? Was the fact that I was still in my pajamas a factor? (Note to self: don't let everything go. Get the fuck dressed.) Was he just busy and I am just overly sensitive?

The latter is no doubt true. For all their sameness my days have their ups and downs. I go for long walks. I have lazy days where I just watch *Outlander* and *Madam Secretary* and *Dead to Me*. I put off washing my hair, again. I am careful with my wine intake, mostly. And food intake, mostly. I cook, then I stop liking cooking. I give up carbs, then welcome them back. I feel my age. I rediscover ice cream. I see my gray hairs. I want to make plans. I feel grateful for my health. I am lonely.

The news reports of virus patients dying without their family around them reminds me of a scare I had in an airplane years ago. The pilot attempted to land at the old Denver airport, Stapleton, on a sunny summer day that included the unfortunate weather effect called wind shear. As we lurched toward the ground, dropping with shuddering thuds on the way down, all the passengers turned to tears or prayer or both. The hush was electrifying. As we faced the all-too-real possibility of death, I vacillated between being glad that I was traveling alone, that my family wouldn't die with me, and being terrified to die alone.

Which is better? To be selfish or selfless: the eternal dilemma. Both are normal reactions. We are not perfect beings. Gripping the armrests, tears streaming down our faces, we felt the plane lift. The pilot took us aloft with what appeared to be a couple hundred feet to the runway. We lived to fly another day. And to be blessed with wind shear alerts in cockpits.

In my dream I run across an old friend. I have given her directions to the beach, or somewhere, and I catch up with her there, excited to see her. She is startled by my appearance, and a little cold. What are you doing here, she seems to say. I am ever-so-slightly crushed.

I am human. Personal rejection is a thing. Obviously. Especially when my writing is not going well. When my muse is at my back I don't care what anyone thinks about me. I am in the moment, flying, digging into the subconscious where the stories live. I am alive. Gloriously alive.

But the pandemic has taken the wind out of my sails. I do get some writing done but not enough. I am worried about my elderly mother, and when, and if, I'll get to see her again. I am worried about my husband, my kids, my grandchildren, my sisters, everybody. I tell them nothing will ever be the same, and wonder if that's true. I worry about my friends and when it will be safe to see them, to hug them, to commiserate about these awful times. I worry about their kids.

Worry comes too easily. Heartache seems around every corner. Uncertainty rules. I cry when I watch news reports on television. I try not to watch the news, and fail. I am angry. I am sad.

But this is life. My husband, a doctor, told me years ago that life is a tragedy. He has seen so many lives extinguished. So we live, as best we can, while there is breath. If you're a writer, your life is writing. I don't believe in writer's block. These are always excuses for not writing, if your work is not going well. Many, many excuses. There will always be worries and uncertainty.

Just get back to work, I tell myself. *Everyone deserves a chance to follow their dreams.* Do my characters deserve that chance? Yes. Am I going to provide them that chance? Yes! Yes, I am.

As soon as I finish the laundry.

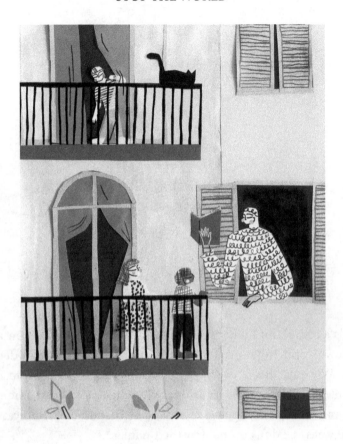

Lise McClendon is the author of 23 novels and numerous short stories. She serves on the faculty of the Jackson Hole Writers Conference and has been a board member of Mystery Writers of America and International Crime Writers Association/North America. She began her career with *The Bluejay Shaman*, set in her home state of Montana, and now writes a series set in France, the **Bennett Sisters Mysteries.** She lives in Montana and California. lisemcclendon.com

MY CROWDED QUARANTINE

BY DAN FESPERMAN

HERE'S a complaint I'll bet you haven't heard much in this new age of lockdowns and isolation: Our house has become too crowded, too noisy. We have been overrun by interloping legions of teachers, reporters, union reps, investors, churchgoers, board members, government officials, spokespersons, and corporate executives. And in many cases, I don't even know their names.

Before you summon the authorities, or suggest cordoning off our house as a super spreader site, let me explain.

My wife, Liz, is a reporter for the *Baltimore Sun*, a newspaper I hold in high regard partly because it once did me the favor of employing me. In March, as lockdown orders went into effect, she began working from home. She also happens to be a union representative at a time of crucial negotiations, a key organizer of a campaign to convince the paper's faraway owners to sell to local interests, a member of her church's governing body, and a partner with her three siblings in an LLC that is renovating and trying to rent an old family home on the Maryland Eastern Shore.

You might say she has a full plate. It is certainly fuller than mine, for whom the main responsibilities are writing novels and teleplays, although the latter are now on hold until conditions permit the resumption of face-to-face writers meetings.

I am long accustomed to working from home, and I have a comfy downstairs office with a panoramic view of the forest bordering our home. Up until March, my average work day was a secluded affair, disturbed only by birdsong. Whenever I got stale, I'd head upstairs with my notes to sprawl on the sunroom couch, or scribble at the kitchen island. I'd break for a sandwich, the crossword, a nap, moving from spot to spot in the proprietary manner of a house cat, daring anyone or anything to disturb me.

I commune with my characters, of course, but they never venture beyond my head, even when nagging at me after hours. If this occurs when you happen to be in the same room, you're none the wiser unless I tell you. Liz occasionally notices my face going blank for a few moments, like the screen of a laptop in need of a reboot, but none of these visitations is intrusive for anyone but me.

Now, many of the spots where I once gravitated for work or lunch are regularly overrun by the long line of participants in Liz's parade of meetings, interviews, strategy sessions, church events and family councils. Their voices carry throughout the house, courtesy of Zoom, FaceTime and the speaker phone function (which keeps her hands free for note-taking). No sooner does an interview end than a union bargaining session begins, followed by a meeting of, say, the Baltimore County School Board, which gives way to a chat with an editor.

I should pause here to acknowledge how lucky we've been to date with regard to the direr consequences of the pandemic. Liz and I are healthy (knock on wood). Our daughter in Brooklyn got the virus in late March, but, other than losing her sense of smell for a week she was not very sick, and she has kept her job. Our son is a graduate student in Montana, which has had so few infections that he's probably likelier to encounter a grizzly bear. Liz and I remain employed. So, ours is not a tragedy, but rather a quirky tale of how life has become much more cloistered yet, in our case, much more cluttered by noisy human interactions.

The peak moment of absurdity was probably the week when, as a union rep, she was negotiating employee furloughs and salary cuts (including hers). Several of these sessions occurred while I was making dinner. Being a former reporter myself, I had a healthy rooting interest. I also happen to be one of those irrational people who often engages in one-way conversations with TV news anchors and sports broadcasters -- "Are you blind? There's no way that was a foul!" But on this occasion I was under strict orders to hold my tongue, since anything I shouted might also be heard by the other participants.

So, there I was, chopping vegetables for the stew pot while Liz sat fifteen feet away, haggling over the newspaper's future. The company's representative began to speak about all of the concessions they wanted, and for me the muttering began.

"Those pricks!" I hissed, as I cleaved a potato with a chef's knife. "That's bullshit," I added a moment later, having moved on to the onions with another mighty whack.

Liz flinched but didn't respond. The company rep then made her case for why any pay cut needed to be permanent, just as I was beheading the green stalks from some carrots.

"Ask why they're trying to reap long term benefits from a short term crisis!" I said, a little too loudly.

"Shh!" Liz hissed over her shoulder.

Chastened, I reached meekly for the celery and tried to tune them out. I set the pot to simmer, and decided that only a shot of bourbon could tide me over to adjournment.

That's the way evenings in our house have often gone lately, with me either eavesdropping on a roomful of virtual visitors or trying to act like they don't exist. A few days ago, when she had taken the latest contingent – the 80 or so members of the union's local – down the hall with her to the spare bedroom, I was reading quietly when I heard the beep of a smoke alarm, chirping for a fresh battery. In the way of all smoke alarms, it did not readily reveal its whereabouts, but the sound seemed to be coming from downstairs. I hustled there and stood, waiting quietly for the next chirp. A faint beep told me that I had miscalculated, so I went back upstairs. The next beep led me down the hallway toward the bedrooms. A minute later I finally realized it was coming from some other home altogether, via the Zoom connection.

It was another hour before the voices finally abated for the evening. Liz and I were once again alone, and it was time for bed.

I turned out the lights and locked the doors. Not that this would do us a damn bit of good. By morning, everyone would start lining up for more, and none of them would need a key for re-entry to our crowded house, our buzzing little beehive of the pandemic.

———

Dan Fesperman's eleven novels of mystery and suspense have won international acclaim, winning the Dashiell Hammett award in the US and two Dagger awards in the UK. A former foreign correspondent for the *Baltimore Sun*, his travels have taken him to three war zones and more than thirty countries. He grew up in North Carolina, graduated from UNC-Chapel Hill, and now lives in Baltimore.

I'D REALLY RATHER NOT

BY KATE FLORA

RECENTLY, I read Melville's *Bartleby the Scrivener*. Bartleby, hired to copy documents in an attorney's office, performs well at first, but then begins to slow down and starts responding to every request his employer makes by saying, "I'd really rather not" until he is doing nothing at all.

Bartleby's response echoes mine as the many weeks of quarantine have passed.

In the beginning, it seemed that a writer's life in quarantine would not be so different from life at all other times. We write. We write some more. Then we write even more. I, and many writers I know, are not particularly social beings, so being shut up at home didn't seem like it was going to be difficult.

I was wrong. It proved to be surprisingly difficult. There was the matter of lack of choice: it is easy to be isolated with the isolation stems from the joy of writing undisturbed. When stories are flowing. Imagination bubbles. Fascinating characters and unexpected scenes and surprises keep appearing. When that isolation becomes enforced, something unexpected happens. The world that was so easy to shut out in normal times finds its way through the cracks and crannies until it becomes an almost unstoppable distraction. What are today's numbers? How many new cases, new deaths, new tests conducted? Have we flattened the curve? When will it end? When will it be safe to get a haircut? Buy groceries in any form other than masked and gloved at a breakneck race during senior hour, refusing to return for anything forgotten on the first pass?

The news has always been there, accessible with a few key clicks, but easy to ignore. That's not the case when you live in a hot zone. I began the days of burgeoning virus in Florida, where I could hear people next door loudly discussing how it was a hoax. I could cycle past groups not observing social distance, and, while the beach parking lots were closed, there were still people on the beach and chatty, indifferent groups blocking the narrow path to the beach. Scarier, though, was the way it was exploding back up north. Was it safe to drive home? Would it even be possible? Would there be restaurants? Hotels? Rest stops? The journey north was us, trucks, and Canadian snowbirds fleeing north before the border closed. There was an unrelenting sense of panic about the journey.

Back home, surrounded by conflicting information, even getting groceries seemed too dangerous. I am over seventy with an under-lying condition. Soon I had a headache. Sore throat. Cough. Was convinced I was definitely going to die. I began reading about Swedish Death Cleaning. I arranged my files so the family could find my insurance policies. I laid in a generous supply of bourbon. In the small office where I've worked for over thirty years, I became unable to concentrate, overwhelmed by the books, the papers, the clutter.

A book deadline loomed and I was so distracted I had no idea what the book was even about. I would tell people I was writing a book where there had been a near death, an attempted murder, attempted arson, a kidnapping, and yet nothing had really happened. I tried to figure out why I was so distracted when life really wasn't different. I found myself increasingly looking at the tasks of daily life —make the bed, clean, do the laundry, wash my hair, bother to get dressed, fix dinner, etc.—and echoing Bartleby. I'd really rather not.

The unproductive days in world of doom and gloom were leav-ened by Zooming. Zoom book events. Zoom cocktail parties. Zoom check-ins with friends. The days began to be punctuated by Zooming in the way they'd been punctuated by real life events. I could look at my calendar and see that instead of speaking at a conference I was zooming with someone. On another day, a favorite library event was replaced by Zooming.

As the Zooms piled up, I found myself responding to those events with my new Bartleby mantra: I'd really rather not.

There had never been enough time to truly get the gardens in order and now I had that time. But after a month on my hands and knees, weeding and digging up plants and succumbing to pictures in flower porn catalogues and buying things I had no place to plant, I was Bartleby again. Roses need fertilizer? Foxgloves need planting? Shrubs pruned? Decorative patio pots need to be filled? Oh Bartleby! I don't wanna.

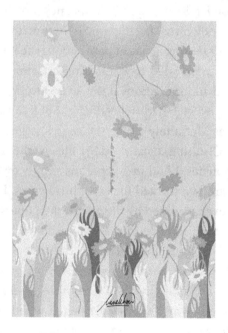

I am sure that the quick answer to me, and Mr. Bartleby, must be that we are depressed. We need to get some exercise, go for a walk (wearing our masks, of course) or we need a little chemical aid to get us through or we should allow ourselves to enjoy cocktail hour more often or we should be grateful that we don't have jobs to worry about (other than the book that's due soon) and we have enough money saved and we have no rent or mortgage due. But with the world of germs hovering just outside the door like an enormous black cloud and people starting to pride themselves on not wearing masks, I don't want to feel grateful or comforted.

For now, I will stare at the blank screen, knowing I must write a thousand words today before I have to go and fix a meal and that this day will be just like the others. I am not in England, walking Hadrian's Wall, and soon on my way to France, as the calendar says. I am frustrated by the state of the world, the way the news makes me feel helpless, and like many others, resentful that this mess has been handled so badly. I am tired of debates over whether to wear a mask. Tired of the newspaper's charts. Tired of trying to be productive and cheerful.

I'd really rather not be.

———

KATE FLORA IS the author of 21 books in fiction, true crime, nonfiction, and short fiction. She's been an editor and a publisher, international president of Sisters in Crime, and a founding member of the New England Crimebake and Maine Crime Wave conferences and runs the Maine Crime Writers blog. She's been a finalist for the Edgar, Anthony, Agatha and Derringer awards, won the Public Safety Writers Award and twice won the Maine Literary Award for Crime Fiction. She's an enthusiastic gardener with a brown thumb and excels at burning rice. Flora divides her time between Maine and Massachusetts and dreams of being a torch singer though she sings like a frog. www.kateclarkflora.com

22

READING BOOKS... OR NOT

BY MARIAN STANLEY

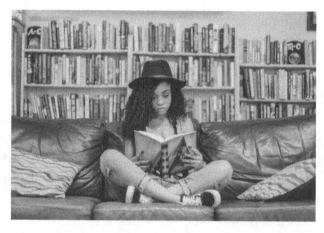

Courtesy Seven Shooter

SOME PEOPLE HAVE difficulty reading and concentrating during this devastating pandemic. I'm familiar with that frustration. The coronavirus occupies too much space in our minds to allow for anything else sometimes.

I experienced the inability to read books – newspapers, yes – books, no – for almost a year after I had a concussion and my husband – whom we care for at home — descended further into

Alzheimer's, all while we had major construction underway and a series of household disasters. The fact that my small publisher went under during this chaotic time was sad, but almost lost in the noise. Perhaps the event was not relevant anyway, since not only was I unable to read books, but apparently I was unable to write one.

Of course, not being able to read or write books was a terrible loss for me. Yet, as we have to do so often in life, I had to adjust to this new reality of the moment – pull up my socks, as they say, and get on with things, which seemed to get more challenging by the week. I think I've done a pretty good job, considering.

Then, a curious thing happened as this pandemic started to engulf us and the number of obituary pages in the Boston Globe began increasing to mind-numbing levels.

One day, shortly after we enter shutdown - huddled in our houses, surrounded by fear, confusion and true heroics - I open a brown cardboard box stashed behind the couch in the parlor. Inside, a draft of the book I was writing when I had my concussion. The book I had stopped dead on last year.

It takes effort at first to focus and read the story through. Even so, I can see that this is basically a good story that needs more work, maybe a restructuring. Slowly, I start to take the book apart. I enlist beta readers, clean the prose up and send the manuscript to a good editor, who I hope is going to help set the book on a better path.

About the same time, someone mentions an interesting biography of Beatrix Potter to me. As an act of faith, since this is a long, dense book and I haven't read a book— other than my own unfinished manuscript— for almost a year, I order a copy from our local bookstore. Maybe I could read a chapter every night and escape into the nineteenth century Lake District. After all, like my own book, which no longer has a publisher, there is no deadline. No need to hurry.

Somehow, while our world is in this strange, apocalyptic coronavirus mode, I am also motivated to dig out, with help, the toxic dump that is our garage after our recent construction. Following that, I tackle the basement, which an environmental team has cleaned up beautifully after a bad backup (see major household disasters above), but left in a jumble.

It will take time and reflection to figure out why the reading and writing part of my brain is suddenly working again and why my capacity for large, physically demanding projects is increasing— both developments just as a worldwide pandemic takes hold. Maybe the scope of the coronavirus plague so vastly overshadows events in my own small world that it is resetting me.

We see our grandchildren on FaceTime and during socially distanced visits. Not quite the same, but very helpful and sweet. Everything about their development seems accelerated— how could they possibly have grown so tall in two months?

Our daughter does most of the shopping and errands for us. We know how fortunate we are. Staying at home in comfort while the storm of the virus swirls around us.

Still, lockdown or not, family support and progress on projects notwithstanding, things happen when someone in the house has dementia. You might leave the key in the door after picking up the newspaper, and realize too late that he's gone. Then, you ride through eerily empty streets, searching for an elderly man in a green checkered flannel shirt, shuffling energetically to a destination mysterious even to himself. Just before you call the police to issue a community alert, your daughter finds your husband in an aisle at CVS, some blocks away. He's forgotten why he went there, but is persuaded, with some difficulty, to come home for lunch.

His morning care program is closed for the duration. Instead, we've settled into a routine of my working around the house in the morning while he reads— or rereads— and watches nature videos. Afternoons, I take him for a ride. The ride, with music on and windows open, is soothing and important for him.

The dog comes along, sitting in a grandchild's car seat. We drive west to towns with farms, orchards and town forests. Usually, we stop for a very short, slow walk. Later, there is ice cream.

If I am burned out and haven't had a chance to rest, the rides and walks– while beautiful– can be draining. This day, when we stop at a peaceful town forest, I am tired and wired from a busy morning.

My husband struggles to open his car door. The dog scrambles to get out, catching his leash in the child seat. Meanwhile, my husband extracts himself from the car. He starts to meander unsteadily toward the forest path which is uneven with raised roots. He doesn't hear or chooses not to hear my call for him to wait.

I never cry. I don't know why that is, but there we are. If I did cry, this might be a time that I do. The enormity of it all. It's too much. Too, too much. But I don't cry.

I catch up with my husband, despite the dog's pulling me back with his leash, wanting to stop at every tree. I take my husband's arm to help him balance. We step into the town forest, quiet and deserted today. The air is fresh. The dog is snuffling happily in the pine needles. And it's okay.

For now, it's okay.

———

MARIAN MCMAHON STANLEY enjoyed a long international career and, most recently, a second at a large urban university. A dual citizen of the United States and Ireland, she lives outside Boston with her husband Bill and a Westie named Archie. She is the author of two Rosaria O'Reilly mysteries *The Immaculate* and *Buried Troubles*, as well as a number of short stories.

ODE ON AMERICAN TP

ALLEN MORRIS JONES

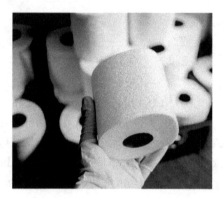

courtesy Erik McLean

We were talking about toilet paper
and I said how I'd like to shake the hand
of the crafty man who invented it.
Such a deceptively ingenious roll
of soft wood pulp, tender enough
to caress but tough enough to do the job
right, humble in its presentation,
waiting patiently for an absent-minded

hand to scroll through, to release
five six eight sheets for a quick crumple
and wipe, tough but fragile, and delicate
enough to dissolve on its way down
the pipe. It's the embodiment of civilization,
if you ask me, utility meets self-indulgence.
"So much we take for granted," I said,
"going about our days without so much
as a second..." And then I noticed
her expression: "What?" She said, "Are
you okay?" I went to the sink to think
about it, washing with soap, happy
birthday twice. "But still," I said.
"Toilet paper."

ALLEN MORRIS JONES is the Spur Award-winning author of the novels *Sweeney on the Rocks, A Bloom of Bones*, and *Last Year's River,* as well as a nonfiction consideration of the ethics of hunting, *A Quiet Place of Violence*, and a children's book, *Montana for Kids: The Story of Our State*. He lives in Bozeman, Montana, with his wife and young son.

A PASS

BY KEITH SNYDER

Skinny bald-headed
oldish guy, strutting like a
banty rooster, arms

out some from his sides,
like that fools any of us
(tallish, though), no mask,

laughs at the paper
signs marking off each six feet
at the pizza place

which is also a
laugh at my mask. I'm walking
back from the drop point

for PPE parts,
I outmass him, mask and shades,
and I give no shit,

am, in fact, minding
my business but feeling mean,
after nine weeks with

no family, no
human touch, just face shields, the
printer clunk and whine.

One doctor's fingers
did brush mine when I handed
him a box of shields—

I still feel it, like
we were lovers. I give the
smug face nothing, stare

at it straight, don't break
stride: damn right, you go around.
Pointless victory
but one asshole down.

KEITH SNYDER'S SHORT STORY, "Blue Skies," appears in issue 5 of Black Cat Mystery Magazine.

PART V

FICTION INSPIRED BY THE PANDEMIC

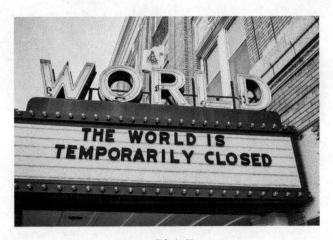

courtesy Edwin Hooper

23

DAY 13
BY RICHARD CASS

IT WAS the gas that did me in, finally. Not the propane, but methane. By Day 11, all I had to do was see him shift in his chair or puff out his cheeks to know what was coming. Eructation. Gaseous eruption. Belch. Funny, I hadn't noticed it much before we were married or even after. One or the other of us was always working, shopping, going to the gym. Doing things. We slept in the same bed, of course, but well, how much did you hear when you were asleep?

But with the entire building on a fourteen-day quarantine, thanks to the mail carrier who'd flown back from Florida in March and returned to work despite a cough and a sore throat, we'd been stuck together in this one bedroom apartment a little too long.

Derek didn't seem to mind the enforced inactivity all that much, which was another thing that irked me. He had beer, chips, and the monocular he used to take on birding expeditions, which he used to spy out our apartment's front window on the building directly across the avenue, a six-story low rise with four apartments on each floor.

"I've seen this movie," I said on Day 6, when he first set it up. I caught a pink flash of flesh at an uncurtained window on the fifth floor, second in on the right.

"No. It's not like the movie at all. I don't have a broken leg, there's no courtyard out there, and we don't live in the kind of neighborhood where people murder their spouses."

"It's creepy," I said. "Voyeur's not a good look on you."

"Ah." He adjusted the tripod and cracked off a belch that bolted up my last frayed nerve. "It's harmless."

I tried not to think about what he'd said, about it not being like the movie, but the idea stuck like a burr to a wool sock.

I kept up with my yoga online. Derek had been a dedicated gym rat before, a lifter, but he was uninterested now in trying to maintain any muscle tone. It surprised me how fast his muscle melted into a puddle of suet. It didn't make him any more desirable.

I burned out on sex by Day 3. He wasn't up to more than one session, and then there was the familiarity factor. Over familiarity, to be honest. Day 8, I started wondering how I was supposed to be faithful to this one man, this body, when this was all over. When I was fifty, sixty, seventy, and still ready to go. This hadn't even lasted two weeks.

He maintained the peeping habit, setting up in the living room every night after dark, all the lights off, beer and bag of chips on the tray table beside him. I moved into the air-conditioned bedroom with my laptop so I didn't have to sit next to him in the dark and listen to him crunch his snacks. They made so much noise it was like his head was hollow.

What set me off finally was the night he strolled into the bedroom, where I'd been watching a documentary on Smokey Robinson and the Miracles, jumped up on the bed, and started kissing me like I'd been out of town for a month.

"Eww." I pushed him off. "Where's that coming from?"

"Nothing." He pouted. "Just trying to start a little something. You've been kind of distant."

"You were trying to suck my tongue out," I said. "Wait! What did you just see out there? You saw something, didn't you? That got you hot and bothered."

He ducked his head the way he did when I caught him out. I could almost wish he was a better liar.

"So what if I did?" he said. "I was only trying to spice up our life a little."

When I saw the Hitchcock movie, I always sympathized more with the Grace Kelly character, the poor woman stuck waiting on the insufferable Jeff. One lousy broken leg and he couldn't do a goddamned thing for himself. Poor woman had been hornswoggled.

If I'd written the movie, maybe Grace Kelly would have snapped at Jeff's whining ways and murdered him, hidden his body. He didn't seem to have too many other friends, anyone else who gave a shit whether he disappeared. I could imagine Grace snapping and skulling him with a frying pan.

I was bored enough with quarantine to wish I had the talent to write it, turn the idea into a story. Maybe it would become a feminist icon, make me famous.

Day 12 eased us up a little, maybe because the end was in sight. The stay-at-home orders were lifting here and there across the state, governed mostly by how many of the lunatic fringe lived in your town. But Day 13 dawned like a garbage fire, hot and humid and rank with the pollution that somehow still hung over the city like an evil fog.

By nightfall, I was sweaty, irritable, and disinclined to do anything but drink cold water and run washcloths over my face and shoulders.

Derek got out his monocular.

"Jesus, Derek. Leave the people alone. It's like you never saw a naked woman."

He lifted his butt cheek and cut a resonant fart. I shook my head, already firm in my desire to leave him. The quarantine had only exposed what an asshole he was.

"Whoa," he said, coming half off the couch.

I looked past his shoulder. A young redheaded woman I'd seen at the farmer's market, talked to in the coffee shop next door, showed in the lighted window of her apartment, sweat gleaming off her pale creamy skin. She stood in front of a fan in an abbreviated pair of underpants.

"You sleaze," I said.

Derek worked up a belch and let it fly, reached for his beer without taking his eye from the monocular. I fantasized hitting the front end of the instrument so hard it would take out his eye.

"Whoa," he moaned, again.

I yanked the power cord free of my laptop, looped it over his head, and pulled as hard as I could. Even harder.

Derek croaked satisfyingly, prying with his hands at the cord, but my rage was too strong for him and slowly, his energy, his life, ebbed and died. I panted, bathed in hot greasy sweat, but when he gasped the last time and slumped forward, I felt exalted, clean, stripped free.

I looked across the avenue at the nearly naked woman, whose eyes were closed as the fan blew air across her breasts. Then one floor above her, I saw the wink of light reflected in a pair of binoculars, the lenses trained down on my apartment. As calmly as I could, I crossed the rug, past the smelly flaccid body of Derek, and pulled the curtain closed. There wouldn't be cool air from the front window any time soon, but I could always be comfortable in the rear.

———

RICHARD CASS IS the author of the Elder Darrow jazz mystery series, the story of an alcoholic who buys a dive bar in Boston, hoping it will help him get sober. The first book in the series, *In Solo Time*, won the Maine Literary Award for Crime Fiction. The fifth title, *Sweetie Bogan's Sorrow*, will be published in September 2020. He's also the author of a book of short stories called *Gleam of Bone*. Cass lives and writes in Cape Elizabeth, ME.

24

NO ROOM! NO ROOM!

BY GARY PHILLIPS

MY GOD. When was the last time she was on a bus, hanging by the strap and not overpowered by someone else's body odor or worse— someone trying to mask their funk with way too much perfume or cologne? Six months ago? Could that be? Had it only been six months since becoming the way things were now? How much longer? Sailors on a carrier or submarine got shore leave. There was no leave from this – at least none was forthcoming. Trials to develop a vaccine had yielded little and estimates for the creation of such were in the years not months.

Katie Claremont had to pause to remember a time when it was safe to bathe and it was fine, even preferred, to have one's own space as they used to say. Huh, when was that phrase last uttered? Probably every damn hour of every damn day she figured as she scanned the faces of the other miserable passengers.

The disembodied voice of the self-driving vehicle announced her stop. Claremont reached past an older woman to pull the signal cord. The woman hacked into her face and smiled sheepishly at the younger woman as several more phlegmy coughs escaped her infected torso.

"Sorry," she said.

"No worries. At least I got it for free."

There were many who subscribed to the theory the more you exposed your body to germs, the better off you were in preventing the onslaught of the virus nicknamed Crowdus. Thus the laxness in washing. There were even cough parties where guests drank or got high and laughing uproariously, coughing on each other. Needless to say, mud wrestling had come back big, for both men and woman and mixed matches as well. Televised events of eight or more tag teaming in the muck had gone through the roof ratings-wise.

Unlike any other time in the history of humankind and pandemics, this particular virus demanded a kind of ongoing herd immunity as opposed to social distancing. As far as the scientists could discern, it was part of delaying the body's natural adaptive immune response that was a factor in preventing the disease. At first the translation of that for people meant they could go about their daily lives, eat in a restaurant, go to the movies or a concert and what have you. You'd be around people. But the virus mutated and as deaths of those in rural areas or families of less than six in an apartment or house mounted, the idea took hold that the more you were around others, the better your chances of not contracting the invisible killer. Not that everyone died from getting the disease. But the effects of having Crowdus were so excruciating, often leaving the patient with various chronic illnesses, folks of course wanted to avoid the risk as much as possible.

Claremont stopped at her neighborhood market to buy a few items. This time of the afternoon, the line was only half way down the block. As was the new normal, people tended to push together a bit more than what would have been acceptable in the past. You might peel away because you wanted semi-privacy while talking on your phone, but the fear was such that arguments and fist fights sometimes broke out if you did this.

"You too good for the rest of us?" would go a typical refrain. "Get your ass back here."

There were too many documented cases when a loner was away from others for more than twenty minutes and when they came back, they had become asymptomatic carriers. The constant pressure was to not be six feet away from other warm bodies. There were some who took to living in isolation gear, essentially modified hazmat suits, but you had to develop a certain mind-set to essentially be enclosed in cumbersome attire pretty much 24/7. As to being intimate, well the word quickie never meant so much as it did now. Orgy clubs had taken on a weird respectability as never before. The open stall, with only a cubicle type wall between the toilets, had become quite the feature. Sleeping arrangements had taken on similar design, with a row of futons separated by a wall a typical layout in mandatory communal living.

The need of keeping others around you constantly had an effect on personal conveyances. Public transportation was way up. For those in their own vehicles, ride-sharing took place in autonomous vans. Deliveries were mostly by drone and long haul trucks had for some time been driverless. Warehouses where orders were filled were always bustling and burnout was common. But there were plenty willing to replace the ones who quit as fulfillment jobs paid well given the necessity of the work. The internet billionaires weren't willingly paying these salaries. But the fact that workers were always huddled together led to so many instances of sabotage, a living wage and humane conditions were the obvious solutions to labor strife. Claremont worked in one such facility.

"Hey, Bill," she said to a lanky man with sad eyes who stepped out the door of her apartment building.

"Right on time," he said as he gave her a half wave and walked off down the street, surrounded by strangers.

Bill was one of her roommates and timing was everything. If one of them had to leave for work, then one of the other seven better be stepping back in. Various staggered and stacked work schedules had to be rigorously maintained. If an accident happened or a bus broke down, then you had to call to tell all concerned.

Entering her apartment, Claremont involuntarily did a quick head count, noting only four of her roommates were in their shared living space. Two of them were watching or listening on their phones, earbuds in, another watching TV with his headphones on and the fourth reading in the corner. None were more than four feet apart.

"Is Meredith here?" she asked, putting away the groceries. Then before anyone could answer, she heard the comforting flush coming from the bathroom. As this was an old building, the john had been designed with a shower, sink and toilet. On the wall was a countdown device and each time an occupant was in there, the timer had an electronic voice warning the user of five minutes left...three minutes and so on.

One time one of them had come back drunk from a co-worker's going away party and passed out on the toilet. Fortunately the timer operated manually or by sensor. Claremont had rushed in there as the robot voice boomed "Alert, Alert, Alert" and shook her roommate awake and dragged the woozy woman to bed to sleep it off.

Meredith came into the room. "Hi, Katie." She plopped down on her usual spot and opened her laptop.

"Hey," she said, trying to sound amiable.

Standing there, the familiar ambiance of being around people who were doing their best to tune out the need to be as close to others as was necessary, made the skin on the back of her neck itch. What was it about the last few days that had gotten to her? Why was it now she so longed to be on top of a snowy mountain staring at clouds? Hyper cabin fever they called it. Lately every damn burp, yawn, and fart had stretched her nerves to the snapping point. Barefoot Brad picking his Cro-Magnon toes, Lindsey's finger twirling her ponytail over and over and over again and Karen and her gum chewing to relieve stress. Was it any wonder the murder rate had skyrocketed?

She went into the bathroom, unable to catch her breath. Shortness of breath was not one of the symptoms of this virus. She started at her reflection in the mirror and for a moment wondered who the hell that haggard looking woman was staring back at her. She wasn't yet thirty but she looked like her Aunt Jean who was twenty-five years older than she was.

"Shit," she muttered. Claremont resisted the urge to grab a knife form the kitchen and chop off a couple of Brad's prehistoric toes. She did though gather her clean clothes and took a shower, letting the alarm go off as she unhurriedly toweled off. She yelled out to assure her roommates she was stepping out. She got dressed in the hallway, out of sight but in proximity to the others. Thereafter she had little choice but to join the others though beneath her calm facade, she was screaming to be alone.

That evening she slept in her clothes. Her cubicle was the last toward the rear and no one noticed. If they had, they would have known what she was going to do. She was about to 'go country,' as it was called.

Early in the dark of morning, Claremont slipped on her moccasins and eased out the back door. She'd greased the hinges a week ago in preparation for this time. Bill was back from work so there were six left in the room. Even at this time of the day there were plenty of people out on the streets. No one paid any attention to her as she walked until the pedestrians began to thin. She wound her way into the industrial area where the robot trucks moved about. There were clusters of humans here but they were in control towers over-looking this vast expanse of asphalt as the 18 wheelers, bobtails, pilot-less forklifts, and logistics drones hummed. A lone figure she knew would show up on their sensors but she wasn't going to be deterred. On she went. High intensity lights snapped on, illuminating her form as two drones buzzed her.

"Miz, please enter the door to your left and come into the control tower." The voice boomed from one of the drones. "You will be imme-diately tested and monitored to make sure you are not infected. Please this is for your safety and ours."

She continued.

"Madam, I implore you to gather with your fellow citizens. Or we will be forced to ask for police assistance."

Her destination was the old 7th Street bridge, a holdover from not only a bygone era, but a bygone century, the 20th. Another warning was issued. She could hear the approach of a police van at her back. She started running. Claremont could see in the near distant mist the snowy peak. She quickened as the van's brakes screeched to a halt behind her and officers alighted from the vehicle. Orders were barked as footfalls got closer. Goddamn LAPD was always in shape.

From over her shoulder a voice said, "Okay, lady, you had your chance."

Electric current shot through her when they blitzed her with a non-lethal compliance weapon. Stars burst behind her eyes and her legs refused to obey. Claremont sank to the ground and was swarmed by bodies in dual protective gear – against germs and bullets. Offering little resistance, she felt the sting of a hypodermic needle piercing her arm. The last thing she saw was that snowy mountaintop. It brought a smile to her face.

THE HYPODERMIC WAS WITHDRAWN, momentarily held upright at the end of the care android's arm. It was then placed back upon a tray that slid back into the control booth where the medical techs looked on. Katie Claremont's withered body lay on the hospital bed in the comforting quarantine room. The drug in her veins did its work and she soon succumbed, fading away like smoke. The plague had ravaged the world, killing tens of millions even though all the precautions had been taken. The result was economic upheaval that resulted in full employment for those left and a green terrain resplendent with animal life and pollinating bees. Katie Claremont's nude body, the brain harvested and a permanent smile on her wrinkled features, was gently carried by the asexual android and placed in a sort of open wicker casket.

These organic coffins were part of a series of conveyor belts at different levels in a vast room where other women and men, also dead and also unclothed, were carried away. The dead were transported to a large brass double door that swung outward allowing them into a processing plant tended by robots overseen by humans. This was where they were ground up in enormous geared teeth. The human mulch would eventually be added to a nitrogen rich mixture and used to fertilize this verdant world, dispensed in industrial-sized bags under the brand called Nature's Gold. Projections were the planet would be down three and a half to four billion before this particular virus was done with destroying the flesh. The remaining population would be heirs to an Earth of incredible colors and smells and a lushness not envisioned since the Garden of Eden.

IN THE OVERCROWDED HOLDING CELL, Katie Claremont awoke, the other narrative already eluding her. A palpable funk assailed her as the women jammed in here tried to assume a comfortable position as there was no room to even sit on the floor. Some managed to sleep standing up. She wished she could do that. At various intervals a voice would announce over the PA system last names first. Those persons would wade through the sea of the arrested and be taken out by the guards as the gate swung open. Claremont was eventually summoned and she went out, escorted along with several others toward the large brass double doors.

————

GARY PHILLIPS WRITES anything he can get away with. His latest is a novel wherein real life North Pole explorer Matthew Henson is reimagined as a pulp adventurer in the Indiana Jones mold, set in the Roaring '20s: *Matthew Henson and the Ice Temple of Harlem*. He lives in Los Angeles.

25

DIAMETRIC AMERICA
BY TRAVIS RICHARDSON

THE NURSE

Exhausting shifts. Then a PPE shortage. N95s long gone. One surgical mask per day. Patients lined up, hacking. Lungs shredded like shrapnel from a grenade. The president says everybody's getting tested. They're not. Dying people gasp through ventilators. They won't make it. Most waiting for one won't either. My colleagues Trish and Mark caught it. They're quarantined. I hate being home feeling useless. Trying to sleep with the images of dead patients painted inside my eyelids. Got to keep working. Save lives. It's what I was born to do.

THE "PATRIOT"

Fuckin' Democrats. They wanna take the vote away from the people. The people who were making America great again. They'll tank the economy so that the president won't get reelected. Total jealousy. Them and the liberal media hate hard working Americans. So do scientists. They've always had it in for capitalism with their environmental hoaxes.

Now they created BS fake news with this Wuhan-Chinese virus

(oops was I not supposed to say that? Sorry not-sorry, Politically Correct Officer.) Ain't no worse than the flu. Limbaugh-Hannity-Ingraham-Dobbs know it. So do Levin, Beck, and Jones. All true red-meat-lovin' Americans. People die from the flu every year, but now we've got to shut down the economy because that's what Pelosi, Biden, Bernie and their brainwashed followers want.

Well, I call bullshit. The cure can't be worse than the disease. Period. Open America up for business, baby. We can handle a freakin' cold. Seriously, folks.

The Nurse

I can't believe these morons. Don't they know what they're doing? People are dying by the hundreds. The morgue can't keep up with the bodies. Regular Americans who were alive and healthy a month ago are dead because they shared space with an infected person. Just when it looked like the curve might flatten, these lunatics—waving flags and carrying guns—want to make America dangerous again.

They say public health experts were wrong, not giving the slightest shred of credit to social distancing. A freakin' effective plan. If the government could organize contact tracing, maybe this virus could get contained and these idiots can go bowling and get tattoos or whatever they so desperately need. But no. Stupidity breeds stupidity. These morons—most without masks—are protesting. I cannot handle it. I must do something.

The "Patriot"

Hell yeah. We're showing them. There's gotta be four-to-five hundred of us real Americans here today. Heck, maybe a thousand. We're strong and proud, while the rest of them sheep stay cooped up inside their houses living under the thumb of tyranny. I've got my Bushmaster Carbon-15 strapped across my chest and my red MAGA hat. You know what I don't have? A mask. Masks are for pussies. I've been working for 30 years and never once had a "legitimate" sick day.

(Deer season don't count.) So come talk to me in your hazmat suit, you commie governor. Me and my friends got a few words for you. And in case you're hard of hearin', I can do sign language. I got a middle finger on each hand.

THE NURSE

My colleagues don't want me to go. They say it doesn't matter; the idiots are too stubborn to listen to reason. But I must do something. Doing nothing is like condoning murder or letting a suicidal patient play with knives. Our silence is killing me. They prance around like their lives and others don't matter. They cry about freedom, but we're in a pandemic. How about caring for your fellow man? I understand your freedom to die, but freedom to infect others? That's not a right. That's terrorism.

Wearing a mask and scrubs, I stand in front of these screaming men and women. I am scared. Although trembling inside, I will not show fear. I have witnessed death many times. I will not be intimidated.

THE "PATRIOT"

Another day not being allowed to work. Another day I'm protesting. Take that libtards. You better believe I'm going to keep this up until every business in this state opens. Fuck you, Fauci. You too, Bill Gates.

What the hell do we have here? One of those actors dressed up like a nurse. Paid to show up and get on the fake news. Not here, sweetheart. Not on my watch.

THE NURSE

Oh God, who is this bearded man standing inches from my face? No mask of course. He's so pre-diabetes if he doesn't have it already. Red-faced, shouting. Spittle flying. Calling me a fake, a terrorist. Saying how he's on to me. So much hate. All I do is save lives.

I've stood as long as I can. Stood for my family of healthcare workers and the dying. Time to go home. Besides, I've got a full shift tomorrow. But I must say something before I leave.

"If you are sick, I will still take care of you."

THE "PATRIOT"

That little bitch stands there, hands behind her back, acting so superior. So smug. If I weren't a gentleman, I'd punch her face.

"Yeah, right, you little faker. Go on back to your little actor's studio and get your paycheck from Soros. See ya."

THE NURSE

Oh, God, it's him. That man so full of rage. I thought he might kill me. Now he's here. On oxygen. I doubt he's going to make it.

THE "PATRIOT"

I feel awful. Got winded just takin' a whiz. My wife's all squealin' about how I've got the covid and I oughta go to the ER. I've only coughed a little. Totally fine. No way I'm going to no hospital. Ain't like I've got insurance or anything.

Oh shit, it's her. The faker. But she ain't. She's the real deal. So is this virus.

"You hate me?"

"Gonna rub this in my face?"

THE NURSE

His voice barely a whisper. But I make out what he said. I've gotten used to breathless conversations. I shake my head no.

"No. I'm going to take care of you."

. . .

THE PATRIOT

She takes my hand in hers. I cry like a baby.

———

TRAVIS RICHARDSON HAS BEEN a finalist and nominee for the Macavity, Anthony, and Derringer short story awards. He has 2 novellas, LOST IN CLOVER and KEEPING THE RECORD. His short story collection, BLOODSHOT AND BRUISED, came out in late 2018. He lives in Los Angeles with his wife and daughter. http://www.tsrichardson.com

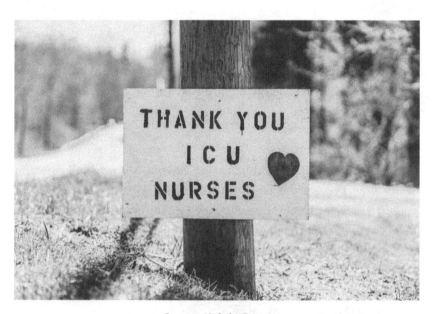

Courtesy Nicholas Bartos

26

ON A HILL NOT TOO FAR
BY JOHN CLARK

HARRY GRIMES TOOK a final hit while watching shadows grow longer in the town below him. *Hope this year's crop is sufficient to get me through all the craziness*, he thought. Like most in Hillman, he hadn't worked since the virus jumped the tracks following a series of ultra-stupid protests at the state capital by mostly poor and desperate folks, goaded by the president's followers. Harry realized well before most did how the exploding case numbers doomed any return to normal, let alone a stable economy.

When you live in the poorest town in the poorest and most conservative county in Maine, you're already behind a couple eight-balls. The Covid-19 pandemic was just the cue stick that shot that third eight-ball into town, shutting the tannery forever. Granted, it had been wobbly for over twenty years, but new owners had come in a decade ago, working with town leaders to gain trust, keeping more than 100 people employed. Now, there was nothing here but desperation.

Hell, with what few people still living in town staying home most of the time, even druggies were having a difficult time getting by. Kinda hard to break in and steal when nobody's ever gone.

If that were the only problem the hundred or so still remaining in town had to face, things might be bearable, but there were others far more dire. The tannery paid 85% of the costs for the water treatment plant. There was no way in hell those remaining could cover the increase in their bills and neither the state or federal government had the interest or resources to step in. Same went for the water company. Just the rental fee for fire hydrants was more than what the town could expect to take in from property taxes now that over half the homes in Hillman were for sale or abandoned. You could also write off the volunteer fire department, the school, the food pantry and the town office.

Those lucky enough to have some form of income but couldn't leave, folks like Ma Grafton his former neighbor who had a disabled husband and two pre-teen grandkids abandoned by their mother a year ago, really struggled. The nearest place to get gas or groceries was in Weston, seven miles away, but potholes were getting worse every time it rained and Harry didn't want to think what would happen when winter hit in a few months. He doubted the roads would be plowed and who knew about propane and heating oil deliveries. Hell, all the things people took for granted two years ago were quickly becoming cosmic rolls of the dice.

Damn good thing I agreed to cabin sit for old man Dempster, Harry thought. The neighbors might creep some people out, but he didn't mind having the Devil's Head cemetery across the road. There were other benefits to living here that far outweighed any unease about the dead. Things like solar panels, gravity fed water and more available firewood than he could cut and burn in ten years. He hoped life was better by then. Either that, or the world might end. He listened to public radio most days, the only news option he trusted any more. Several programs in the past month alluded to mutations of the virus so strong and resistant they were even scaring climate deniers and anti-vaxxers. If half of what the experts were talking about was true, mankind better find a hole, climb in, and hide the entrance.

The last light was fading from Hillman now. Harry knew he shouldn't watch, but there was something so perverse about what would occur in the next few minutes, he couldn't stop his evening ritual.

Everyone knew about the rats living in the tannery. It was a perfect habitat for rodents. They had warmth, the river flowed beside it, there were hundreds of places where they could hide and breed, not to mention all the food dropped by workers. Once the tannery closed, the wily critters had adapted quickly, surviving on discarded leather scraps.

Now those were all gone and the rats came out at dusk to feed. That would have been enough of a nuisance by itself, but environmental factors nobody could have imagined had come into play. Leather is cured with a brine with a very high chromium content. It was not only toxic, but had been linked to at least two cancer clusters in town over the years, both conveniently ignored by citizens because of job security at the tannery.

Rats breed quickly and often. Those about to come out and forage were full of chromium. It had made them bigger, nastier, and a hell of a lot more voracious, but that wasn't what fascinated Harry. No, it was how they glowed with an obscene yellow luminescence when they streamed from the building each night, intent on feeding. Feeding on Harry's former neighbors.

————

JOHN CLARK IS a retired librarian and active book reviewer with a background in mental health. He gardens and continues to write young adult novels as well as short crime and horror stories. He lives with his wife, a retired professor of nursing, in central Maine.

27

COVID LONE RANGER

BY JOHN SHEPPHIRD

"HE WORE a mask like the Lone Ranger," Imran said.

By that point in the lockdown Martina Gomez thought she'd seen it all. She wrote crime stories for the digital news service *Mercury* that covered local and breaking news. The pieces were short, sometimes only two paragraphs. Her beat was the beach cities, south of Los Angeles International Airport and north of the Palos Verdes Peninsula.

The incident had taken place in a strip mall in Torrance. She adjusted her mask, itchy on her face, before she asked Imran, the store owner, "Was his mask disposable or cloth?"

"Rubber, I think," he said. "It wasn't over his mouth and nose like everyone else. It was over the eyes," Imran demonstrated with his fingers, "like the Lone Ranger. And he wore a white hat."

"A cowboy hat?"

"Yes. And boots I think. I have it all on video."

He showed her the surveillance footage. He was a tall guy that appeared to be in his early twenties. From the camera angle the mask was clearly visible. She used her phone to snap a few photos off the monitor, pleased with the results.

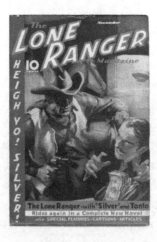

Martina was familiar with the Lone Ranger from old black and white clips on YouTube. And wasn't there a movie with Johnny Depp? She remembered he played the Indian sidekick Tonto instead of the title character. Martina asked Imran, "Did he take anything else other than beer?"

"He came in, grabbed Coors Light and walked out without paying, as you can see. What's strange...he had the music playing on his phone."

"What music?"

"The Lone Ranger music. You know." he hummed a few bars. "You can't hear it in the surveillance video because my security system doesn't record audio."

"The William Tell Overture?"

"The Lone Ranger music, yes," he said. "William Tell."

Even though she found this strangely odd and amusing, there wasn't much of a story here. She tried to imagine what the headline might be.

As much as she resented it, Martina had come to terms with the fact that the stories she wrote for *Mercury* were click-bait journalism. Much like the tabloids, attention-grabbing headlines were key. Martina regretted that she'd majored in journalism. Careers were dying on the vine and she hadn't really started hers, other than the few freelance jobs here and there. Maybe she should have listened to her mother who wanted her to take up a career in nursing instead. At least that was steady.

Martina needed something catchy.

"Do you know who William Tell is?" Imran asked her.

"Refresh my memory."

"He was a Swiss folk hero and expert archer. As the story goes, an oppressive Austrian soldier forced him to shoot an apple off his son's head. Can you imagine? His own son. He had to do it or they'd kill him. So he took aim and nailed it with a single shot. The soldier saw he had a second arrow and asked what that was for. He said, 'If I'd missed and killed my son, the second arrow was for you.'"

"How's that relevant?" Martina asked.

"It's not, but I find it most fascinating." From his accent he was clearly from some Slavic country she couldn't place. "I've had a lot of customers come in lately with bandito scarves across their face but they were very polite and nobody stole anything. Many of them show their appreciation that we're open for business."

"Could someone be playing a prank on you?" Martina asked.

In all seriousness, Imran said, "There's nothing funny about crime." He motioned below the counter. "And if someone tries to rob the cash register...I've got a second arrow like William Tell, if you know what I mean."

Martina took down the information she needed then returned to her car. She peeled off the mask, dug out her laptop and began to write the story. With so much more dramatic news in the cycle, plus Trump, she was doubtful this would ever see the light-of-day. She only got paid if it ran, and since she'd already put effort into it, why not? Either way her editor would decide. But she needed a hook, a headline. It came to her. *Lone Ranger Loots Light Beer* with the subheading *Who Was That Masked Man?*

Martina tethered her laptop to her cell phone and sent it in, certain the fluff piece would never be published. By the time she was back at her apartment she was surprised to see the story online.

The next day she interviewed a Hermosa Beach 7-11 attendant who came across the bandit. Coors Light was clearly his beverage of choice. Her story had an update; her next headline, *Lone Ranger Thief Strikes Again.*

The next day the mysterious thief went into a Ralph's supermarket in Manhattan Beach and on the way out posed with the twelve pack or Coors Light for the surveillance camera at the door. He showed a toothy, sardonic grin and gave the camera a thumbs-up. Martina was able to obtain the image. Her update read, *"Hi-yo Silver Bullet: Lone Ranger Bandit Taunts Authorities."* The cops weren't looking for the guy but it made good click bait.

The story was picked up by news services as a novelty piece. It was shared on social media. Before she knew it, Martina was hearing from old college friends who'd seen her name. She lamented why the stupidest story she'd ever written found traction, while her hard-hitting, world-changing stories went largely unread.

When the demonstrations, riots and looting started that was the end of the COVID Lone Ranger coverage. As far as Martina knew, he never struck again.

Everything had escalated.

Martina knew readers would never know who he was. This was a mystery for the books, kind of like Jack the Ripper, but petty larceny instead of murder.

She came to terms with writing click bait. It was the new normal. And with the Lone Ranger she often wondered: Who was that masked man?

———

JOHN SHEPPHIRD IS a Shamus Award-winning author and writer/director of television movies. Mystery Scene Magazine calls his novel BOTTOM FEEDERS "A fast-paced, fun read that explores a part of the movie business that often gets overlooked... from 'Action!' to 'Cut' it's a pleasure to read." He lives in California. johnshepphird.com

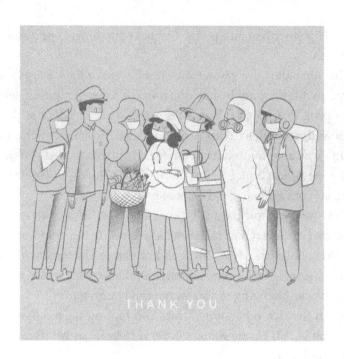

28

PANDEMIC

BY MIKE MONSON

SUNDAY, March 8, 2020.

Went out to drive at 5 am.

As I walked through the parking lot to my car, I noticed the clear sky and large moon.

Clocks had just gone forward, so I knew I was essentially going out into a world that was still, basically, living at 4 am, living in late late late Saturday night.

First several rides reflected the old time — picked up still drunk but exhausted people at Denny's and Jack in the Box and at house parties.

Helped herd them home.

The Lyft app was acting strange— canceling rides that had already started, sending me to destinations rather than the pickup locations, etc. It felt kind of crazy — odd.

About 6:30, I picked up June at a crummy apartment complex off of Paradise Road. She was wearing a large coat — the kind that goes all the way to the knees.

She had two children. A boy and a girl about 8 and 10 or so. They were silent kids. Each wore a black hoodie, and each wore a surgical mask.

I'd heard all the talk about the coronavirus but hadn't paid a lot of attention.

The destination was Doctor's Hospital— about 10 minutes away.

As we drove and as June talked to me, she continually handed each child a wipe from a dispenser, had them wipe their hands, and then placed the used wipes in a white plastic bag.

"I've had pneumonia for three months. I have lupus— the kind that gets in your blood. The bad kind. I don't want to be sick, not now."

As we drove, I noticed more and more people walking— all in the same direction we were going. Some wore masks and some did not.

"I've been doing research for the past 36 hours straight. We are being lied to. They say the infected population here in Northern California is in the dozens but it's actually 80,000 as of midnight and growing.

"Trains and ships and buses full of travelers aren't being quarantined as they claim. They are being dumped in San Francisco and Oakland. They've infected the people who live here and work out there."

Getting closer to the hospital the streets got more and more crowded.

When we pulled up to the hospital, I couldn't drive to the ER entrance because it was surrounded by hundreds of people. Some trying to get in, some trying to get out.

June had me stop so she and her children could exit the car. As my back doors opened, masked men tried to get inside. I had to get out, lock my doors from the outside with the fob, and fight them off.

I finally managed to get back into the car — alone — and drove through the throng and back out into the street.

I headed East toward the mountains.

I have a friend up there who lives off the grid and off the land. He's always trying to get me to come join him "before the world ends" and I always laugh at him.

I hope he still has a place for me.

. . .

MIKE MONSON IS the author of the noir/crime novellas *The Scent of New Death, What Happens in Reno,* and *A Killer's Love,* as well as the crime novel *Tussinland.* He is preparing to publish the book, *Ridesharing,* a collection of fictional stories based on his experiences as an Uber/Lyft driver. He has written a feature movie script based on his novella What Happens in Reno, and is working on a script based on The Scent of New Death (retitled for the screen as Revenge Plot). Also, he is creating scripts for a projected anthology TV series based on the stories in *Ridesharing.* He is a graduate of Chapman University.

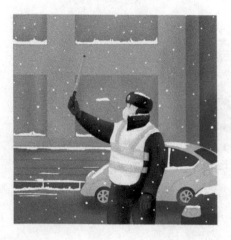

HAIKUS

BY Z.J. CZUPOR

Forget travel plans
Forget eating out with friends
But remember you.

———

Some need PPE
Some need TV and TP
We all need some faith.

———

We hike, bike, and golf
We break our days with Zoom meets
And...we go...nowhere.

———

For whom the bell tolls

For the thousands who have died
Damn! Stop the ringing!

LOCKED IN
BY GERALD SO

Forced home
to stay the past
two months
while essentials
work the newest
breathtaking problem,
I can't imagine
how it's been
for people who
all their lives
have gone out
and moved.
I lost my breath
at hours old,
I'm told,
and since,
have been
behind lazy eyes,
shambling limbs,

the bulk of my ideas
living only on paper.

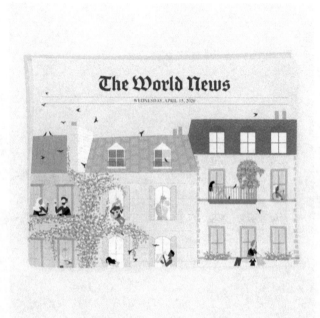

FROM NEW YORK, Gerald So is editor of The Five-Two weekly crime poetry site, new every Monday at http://poemsoncrime.blogspot.com. Follow him on Twitter @g_so.

PART VI

BEYOND THE NOW

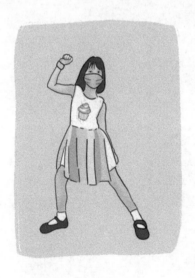

Kate Hourihan

29

FINDING HOPE
BY ROBIN BURCELL

WE CALIFORNIANS HAVE BEEN SHELTERING in place for weeks on end, only emerging for essential business. Today I have a doctor's appointment. Once finished, I head to the other side of town to pick up a letter delivered to the wrong address. Because outings are rare these days, I am taking my time, enjoying the solitude as I sit in my car at a red light. I glance to my left, seeing a utility box on the corner, a bit surprised that I've never noticed the giant dandelion puff painted upon it in black against a yellow-beige background.

The utility box is almost hidden in the dappled shade of a massive redwood tree growing nearby. The painted dandelion tuft is leaning to one side from the force of an invisible breeze wafting against it, the seeds ready to scatter into the world. I almost look away, but my eye catches on a single word hidden within the tuft: HOPE. A vivid, decades-old memory pops into my head of my children picking dandelion puffs from the grass, making a wish, blowing hard, watching the tiny specks of fluff floating through the air.

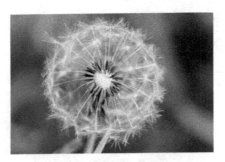

courtesy Griffin Wooldridge

The painted utility box is located directly across the street from a now-shuttered elementary school, where young children used to walk past each day on their way to class. I glance at the empty school then back at the box, reading, embracing the message. HOPE. It's something I need so much right now as my emotions run the gamut with the daily onslaught of news of the pandemic that is not yet loosening its hold on the world. Soon, though, the light turns green. Reluctantly, I let my foot off the brake, edging out into the intersection. As I make a left turn, I crane my neck around, finding a second dandelion tuft painted on the north side of the box, along with another message: BELIEVE.

I am still thinking about that box as I continue down the street to pick up the letter that had been mailed to my former house. In past visits, I'd stop to chat with the owners, who have now lived there a little over two years. But in this new world, as evidenced by the shoes neatly lined up at their front door, the outside is not allowed in, and so I retrieve the letter from below the doormat, get into my car, and leave. Instead of turning right to take the shorter route home, I turn left. I want to drive by that utility box, see it again. I want to know if there is something else painted on one of the other sides.

I slowly cruise past, seeing BELIEVE, then HOPE within their respective dandelions. On the south side, hidden in the tuft is the word WISH. Although I can't see that fourth side of the box, I'm reminded of a favorite scripture and decide the hidden word must be FAITH—which only has to be the size of a mustard seed. Or a dandelion seed, I think, and for the first time in weeks, a sense of calm comes over me as I make my way home.

THIS PIECE *originally appeared in the* **Lodi News Sentinel** *on May 21, 2020.*

———

ROBIN BURCELL, a *New York Times* bestselling author, co-writes the Sam and Remi Fargo Adventures with Clive Cussler. Their latest book, *Wrath of Poseidon*, debuted May 26, 2020. www.RobinBur-cell.com

30

THE UNINVITED GUEST

BY J. MADISON DAVIS

I WAS TWELVE, or maybe just thirteen, sitting alone in about the tenth row of the Cheverly Theater, an old-fashioned movie house with over 500 seats—too many for the business to survive past the 1970s. As the movie began, I was nibbling popcorn greased with that pseudo-butter they use. The feature was *The Masque of the Red Death*, starring that hambone of horror, Vincent Price. Roger Corman, the director, knew to great success that you can't make a good pot of beans without an unrepentant hambone. Corman survived long enough to become a cult figure and acquire a lifetime achievement Oscar, but at the time, who knew? No one mistook these bubbling bean-pots for art. Exploiting the name of Edgar Allan Poe was eight times one of his come-ons, providing a literary cachet which allowed me to cadge the price of admission out of my dad. All I knew was that I enjoyed this stuff. We learn a lot while we're thinking we're just having a good time.

Like most Poe stories, "The Masque of the Red Death" is intense, simple, and pure. Intended to be read in one sitting, it doesn't have enough story for a feature film. To solve this problem, some Poe movies combine two stories, like mashing together "The Black Cat" and "The Cask of Amontillado," but *Masque* was simply padded with some foolishness about the main character (Prince Prospero) lusting after a shapely village woman, provoking the jealousy of his current squeeze, and practicing Satanism. Poe's story is much simpler, but remains intact in the movie despite being padded and stretched. Prospero's dominions are being devastated by the Red Death, a fictional plague. Blood issues from the pores of its victims and they die in quick, painful agony. I understand that sweating blood is sometimes a symptom of arsenic poisoning, but as I say, Poe invented the illness, so it has no parallel in the natural world.

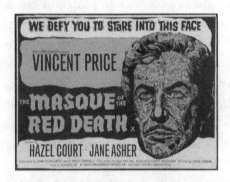

Prospero deals with the plague by inviting a thousand of his noble friends to his remarkable abbey luxuriously described by Poe as having a series of rooms done in a succession of vivid colors. All "the appliances of pleasure" will be provided: clowns, dancers, wine, and (*naturalmente!*) beauteous women. Everyone will be locked in. Outside, the Red Death will go on ravaging the countryside as the peasants go about their business, presumably doing the essential jobs for which they are underpaid at the medieval equivalent of Walmart, and dying in agony.

Prospero, stable genius that he is, prepares a masked ball. Why think about what is going on out there? The partying is hardy until some of the guests begin to notice a tall figure in a corpse-like mask and a ghoulish, blood-spattered costume intended to simulate a victim of the Red Death. Prospero is furious. Who would dare pull such a trick on him? He demands the tall figure be seized and says he will be hanged from the battlements at sunrise. Getting no immediate response, Prospero draws a dagger and raises it over his head, but before he can strike, drops the dagger and dies on the spot. When the guests gather enough courage to seize the intruder, the costume collapses. It is empty. The guests also begin dropping until all of them are dead. In the movie, the shapely girl Prospero abducted survives—*naturalmente!*—along with a handful of sturdy villagers, which kind of misses Poe's point, but hooray for Hollywood.

As all of this transpired, I sat in the tenth row, now eating gingerly. I had begun to feel a certain nausea. I thought maybe it was the pseudo-butter on the popcorn. Then I thought the movie was getting to me by showing so much of the Red Death it was making me think that I actually had it. By that night, my pores were not bleeding, but there was no doubt I was sick. I couldn't keep anything down nor anything in. My mother would splurge on Canada Dry ginger ale when my brothers and I had a fever or intestinal distress and put the ice-filled glasses by the bed. Days passed, however, and I sank further into the sickness. She noticed that I had difficulty getting the glass. I was too weak to pick it up.

In the emergency room, they could not identify what caused my condition, but I was severely dehydrated. They speculated it was some kind of dysentery, but what? The lab work revealed nothing. I was in serious danger. I was given an intravenous drip, and, quite remarkable for those days, a private room. It was a very stark, prison-like room, but until they could identify what the problem was they didn't want me near any other patients. There wasn't even a television in the room, and that didn't matter because I didn't have my glasses and couldn't see anything anyway. I remember the happiness I felt when I heard the keys my father hung around his waist clinking down the hallway looking for my room. I couldn't see him, but I knew he was there. When he entered the room, I was too myopic to see his face or recognize him because they had dressed him in a full white doctor's gown, hat, and mask over his bus driver's uniform.

"Whatcha doing?" he asked, gently resting his hand on the sheet over my thigh.

I pointed to the intravenous fluid. "Having lunch," I said.

Gradually the intravenous fluids began restoring me and the illness subsided. Doctors regularly interrogated me as to what I ate that no one else in my house had eaten. Since I had felt ill just as I began the popcorn, they ruled that out. The only thing I could think of was that I filched a green olive when no one was looking. The doctors all rejected that as being far too salty to carry any pathogens. They asked me if I had to drunk any water out of a puddle. I was a little offended that they would think a person of my advanced age would be drinking out of puddles, and more offended that they wouldn't believe I hadn't.

Finally, they decided whatever I had couldn't be that contagious and the nurse rolled in a television on a cart. There were no remote controls and I had to slither down to the end of the bed rolling my intravenous paraphernalia behind me until I could unsteadily reach out over the footboard and change the channel. The nurse came in one night, and I was still watching television about nine o'clock. She asked me didn't I think it was time for bed and I remember protesting "But we always watch Perry Mason!" She smiled and let me watch it.

Upon my release, I was ordered on a strict no-fat diet for a month or so, and it seemed like, as my innards were healing, all my family ate that month was particularly delicious, but oily foods. They would have steak or fried chicken, and I would have Farina—no milk—or yet another bowl of Campbell's chicken noodle soup. My mother made a chocolate pudding cake, and finally in sympathy of my misery, she froze a good chunk of it for me to eat once the month was over, leading to the discovery that it wasn't the kind of food that freezes well. She broke my no fat-diet regime a few days early with a thin hamburger, broiled and patted with paper towels until it was about as greaseless as a hamburger could be. Prince Prospero's personal chef couldn't have made such a good burger.

What had I survived? I don't know. Nobody knew. Even less did they know why I survived. Most diseases are obvious. Some manifest themselves in peculiar and unpredictable symptoms. You grasp at the garments of the guest you do not recognize, and the costume collapses. The garments are empty and the wearer has disappeared.

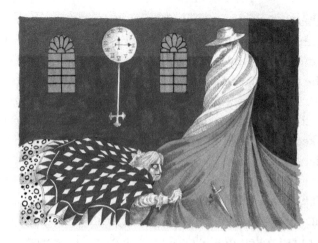

The message of Poe's story and its overwrought film adaptation proved to be an essential statement about this fragile thing we call life. After all, it was the sixties and we were all as Poe describes Prospero: "happy and dauntless and sagacious." Disease was being conquered. Antibiotics had been discovered only a few decades before the movie was made. It hadn't been that long since polio vaccine had been created, and there was no reason to think that the conquest of disease wouldn't lock pestilence forever out of our homes. As a child I had measles, chickenpox, and a mild case of mumps. On my shoulder is the scar from the smallpox vaccination that is no longer necessary. My children have never had measles or chickenpox or whooping cough or mumps or polio or diphtheria, and there is no reason (no good reason!) my children's children should ever have them.

But this pandemic we are currently locked away from in our homes reminds us that the Red Death goes anywhere he wants. As insubstantial as an empty shroud, he randomly appears in costumes many times more various than the rooms in Prospero's abbey. We cannot know what form he will take, dressed in the blood of a flea or a bat or a pangolin or your neighbor's cat. He appears at his own will, indifferent to everything we hate and love. No matter how brilliant we imagine ourselves to be, no matter what our hopes and dreams, with a stare he forces us to drop the pathetic dagger of our arrogance.

As Poe put it:

"And now was acknowledged the presence of The Red Death . . . and Darkness and Decay and the Red Death held illimitable dominion over all."

———

J. Madison Davis is the author of eight novels—several of which were nominated for awards and one of which was briefly an e-book best seller. He has also published seven nonfiction books, and dozens of short stories and articles. He was a columnist on international crime writing for World Literature Today for fifteen years, and is a Professor Emeritus of the University of Oklahoma. In the summer of 2008, he was elected the President of the International Association of Crime Writers, and now lives at Lake Monticello, Virginia.

31

THE MASK

BY MATT COYLE

I WORE a face mask before it was cool.

The virus news out of China in January forced me into Always Be Prepared mode, even though I was never a Boy Scout— in too many ways to count. It took over a month for the mask I ordered on Amazon to arrive. I wore it in Target and got stares, even from the one other person in the store wearing one. I gave the woman a nod and she social distanced times ten away from me.

Then the experts on TV tried to make me feel guilty for wearing a mask because they initially claimed it could do more harm than good. That didn't sound like a very educated expert thing to me. I believe in self-preservation, so I still wore the mask. Turned out the experts were really trying to discourage the public from buying masks that were needed for medical workers. I understood their reasoning, but the experts had breached my trust.

American industry went to work and now everyone has a mask. Or three. You can even make one a fashion statement. For those of us who wear glasses, a mask is just a permanent fog machine. I don't recommend it for driving.

Now you'd better wear a mask the second you leave your house, where most experts claim the virus lives best. Inside. The experts have given us a lot of conflicting advice on the virus, some from the same expert just weeks apart. It's like watching the science in fast motion. What was wrong is now right and what was right is now wrong. Interesting from afar, but a disjointed way to live in practice.

I still listen to the experts and I still wear my mask. But I listen to the common sense within me, too.

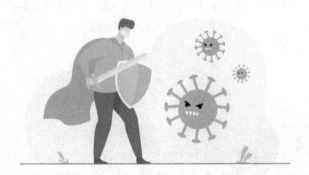

Matt Coyle is the author of the bestselling Rick Cahill crime series. His books have won the Anthony, Lefty, Ben Franklin Silver, Foreword Reviews Book of the Year Silver, and San Diego Book Awards, and have been nominated for the multiple Macavity and Shamus Awards, as well as named to numerous Best Of lists. Matt hosts the Crime Corner podcast on the Authors on the Air Global Radio Network and lives in San Diego with his yellow Lab, Angus, where he is writing his eighth crime novel.

https://mattcoylebooks.com/

32

DEATH IN THE TIME OF CHOLERA
BY SHARAN NEWMAN

THOMAS EDGAR WAS BORN in 1777 in New Jersey, nine months after his father, James, had a weekend pass from the Revolution. Or maybe it was just a quick visit, as the war was going on all around his hometown of Woodbridge, New Jersey. Thomas's mother, Isabelle, died when he was three. The story of how it happened is lost in family legend but the British seem to have been involved. He was raised by a stepmother and grew up in the turmoil of the new nation.

When he was 21, Thomas married Mary Freeman, the daughter of another Revolutionary patriot. Her father wasn't in the army but, as a carter, smuggled guns into British-held New York City. He was captured and put on a prison ship where many died of typhoid. However, his brothers, cousins, and friends wouldn't put up with that and mounted a sea rescue, also the source of many legends.

Thomas and Mary had seven children, three of whom died young. By 1849, they were living on Vandam Avenue in New York City. He gave his occupation as "wood inspector." His pride in life was being an elder in the Spring Street Presbyterian Church, (torn down in 2006 to build Trump Soho.) As a deacon he also inspected people, visiting those whose attendance at church was irregular or lives were immoral. Records show that one woman, chided for her dissolute life, sent the deacon packing with some highly unladylike words.

A normal, if stuffy couple of no particular interest to history, so why write about them? For me it's because they weren't important, merely a statistic. In the winter of 1849, there were thousands of such statistics.

That's when the second wave of cholera hit.

The first cholera epidemic had begun years earlier, in 1832. That year the board of health suggested that there were more deaths than usual, but cautioned people not to panic. *The New York Evening Post* told readers that they shouldn't flee the city, because the panic was invented. They reminded them that most cholera deaths were among people of an "intemperate" nature, drunks and women of ill repute and those "who ate lemons, skins and all."

Of course, if readers had examined the list on the same page, they would have noticed that the victims included two children, ages five and eight, and their mother. It's odd the way the media can print two opposite things and people only believe the one that's an editorial.

The 1832 epidemic followed the waterways. No one knew how cholera spread. Some thought it was airborne, others that it was caused by an excess of electrical charge in the air. There was some thought that unsanitary living conditions exacerbated the illness, but that didn't explain how it seemed to flow into the homes of the wealthy.

Local merchants tried unsuccessfully to calm panic by suppressing information. Cholera was not good for business. Business was depressed. Organized religion thrived. National and state days of prayer were appointed to appease an angry God. One Presbyterian newspaper stated: "We regard cholera as the judgment of God upon a sinful nation, an intemperate, ungrateful Sabbath-breaking nation. a nation which has robbed and spoiled the Indian and withheld that which is just and right from the enslaved African. Cholera will go where it is sent. Best advice: Be ready for death. Death stands at your door. Repent of your sins."

It is not recorded that anyone in power acted upon this advice.

Eventually, the epidemic ebbed and Americans returned to normality. By 1849, the cities had grown, the roads were better, and trains were beginning to appear. "There is clear evidence that the disease entered the United States at two points within a nine-day period of time. New York was attacked on December 2, 1848, and New Orleans felt the first effects on December 11." This time it spread up the Mississippi River as well as through the Great Lakes and the Ohio River.

Attitudes hadn't changed since 1832. It was said that the cholera emanated from the cesspool of the Five Points, an area mostly inhabited by freed slaves and immigrant Irish. Built on landfill the houses had soon sagged. Dickens wrote, "What place is this, to which the squalid street conducts us? A kind of square of leprous houses, some of which are attainable only by crazy wooden stairs without. What lies behind this tottering flight of steps? Let us go on again and plunge into the Five Points."

Thomas and Mary Edgar were not alarmed enough to leave the city. They may have believed that their stalwart Presbyterianism would protect them, aided by one of the many miracle cures advertised in the papers, mainly laudanum, opium, peppermint oil, and a special secret ingredient.

None of them worked. Mary died June 9, 1849, Thomas the next day. They were buried hastily, with no ceremony but a prayer. They weren't interesting or important, except to their family. They were just two of the 400 people who died in New York that week.

We look at the statistics every day. They are just numbers. But each number represents a life, then and now. No one is expendable. The saddest part of this is that, in 170 years, we have learned how to take a virus apart. We have amazing pills and machines to treat it. But faced with an invisible killer, we still hunt for someone to blame and put our trust in miracle cures.

In 1849, in London, John Snow made the connection between water sources and cholera. Clean drinking water is the only way to prevent it. The only 'cure' is still replacing the water and salt that the body is losing. There is no vaccine.

———

SHARAN NEWMAN IS a medieval historian who writes the Catherine Lavender mysteries and also non-fiction. She lives near a village in Ireland with a view of the Shannon Estuary, where people take the supernatural as normal. http://www.sharannewman.com

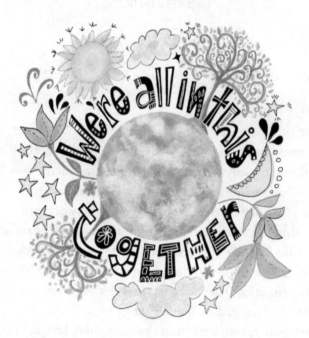

FLIP THE COIN

BY MEREDITH BLEVINS

TWIN BROTHERS STOOD on a dock in Ireland. The year was 1888. They'd moved from the countryside, the youngest two of twelve children, and into the city to earn money for a fresh start. One became a boxer. The other brother brought the folks in and took their bets. After one year, they'd saved enough to make new dreams.

Twin ships were harbored, one bound for New Zealand and the other to Ellis Island. The brothers flipped a coin. Heads, and one boy's destiny was in the southern hemisphere; tails and the other was headed for America. They laughed into the sky from the sheer joy of being alive, and hugged each other tight.

At first glance, they grew into ordinary men. Digging deeper, one founded an orphanage in New Zealand, and the other struggled for worker's rights on the docks in San Francisco. They worked hard, kept dreaming, and raised strong children. Their family tree is filled with ordinary heroes, the best kind.

The man who went to San Francisco, my grandfather, had three children. The oldest two were hit hard by the Spanish flu—both had nerve damage the rest of their lives. Regardless, they all carried on and lived big lives, full of color, tinged with tragedy, and escapades resulting from love with the right people at the wrong time. The stuff of all big lives.

And today I wonder: What lives have been changed because two people couldn't stand on a dock and flip a coin? What babies weren't made during this time of physical distancing? (Because deep kisses, right in the center of the mystery, don't happen over ZOOM.) What art came to life because someone finally made time to go inside themselves and create beauty? When noticing that we, in fact, might be mortal, how many of us decided to be fully alive, no holds barred, until we checked out of Hotel Earth?

What an extraordinary future that bold decision will shape.

———

MEREDITH BLEVINS IS the author of seven novels for Macmillan, and one non-fiction for Rodale. She has a new story in the works and is also a travel writer. Her life has been filled with bold women who turned their backs on the color beige. The Southwest is home for Meredith and her husband, author Win Blevins. For more: www.prowriterstoolbox.com

BEHOLD THE TAKE-OUT MENU
BY JIM NISBET

News hath no harridan
Like Brent Crude Presents
Not even serological probity
  Can score a dent

Upon its carapace of perfidy
  Nor dis-embitter its blonde
Cocktail of bile, a caravansary of ignorance
  Tuned to an oligarch's smile.

A gluteus osculated as regular
  As a walking beam pumps,
No demeanor too sedulous
  Only muck to cloy the sump

Of conscience, neutrino smiles,
 A mien devoid of meaning
A Moloch never brought to Barr

While all the world is teeming

With millepædal Corporations
And their vile suppurations

High time to spear their writhing convolutions
  Upon the pitted tines of pitiless Revolution
Else it's back to sleep with you, jobless
Proletariat,
  Strangled to dreamless Purgatory

By Kapital's coarse lariat.

JIM NISBET HAS PUBLISHED twenty books: thirteen novels including *Lethal Injection*, a classic roman noir, six volumes of poetry, and a nonfiction title, *Laminating The Conic Frustum*. He is at work on two more novels, a complete translation of Charles Baudelaire's *Les Fleurs du Mal*, and a growing collection of Plague Ditties. He lives in the Bay Area, California.

  http://noirconeville.com/

HAIKUS

BY Z.J. CZUPOR

The hum of highway
Is like the life we live now
Quiet, Gone, Uncertain.

———

Slow down, don't move fast.
Gotta make the virus pass.
Screw it! Pass the scotch.

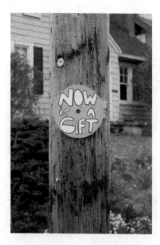

courtesy Zachary Keimig

Let's play whack-a-mole
Stop the virus forever.
There it is. No. There.

———

Let's kill the virus.
Let's murder its pathogen.
Who would convict us?

———

Z.J. CZUPOR LIVES IN DENVER with his wife and two rescued collies. He writes a monthly column, The Mystery Minute, for the Rocky Mountain Chapter Mystery Writers of America. They can be found at www.rmmwa.org. Since the coronavirus pandemic started, Z.J. began writing and posting poetry on Facebook in the form of haikus, called "Today's Noir Haiku." Follow the entire thread at www. facebook.com/zjczupor.

ABOUT THE CONTRIBUTORS

GEORGE ARION is a Romanian journalist famous for his interviews and also an author who writes multiple literary genres - poetry, prose, drama and essays. He is the author of movie and TV scripts, as well as of an opera libretto. He has been thrice awarded with The Romanian Writers' Union prize and also with the Romanian Writers' Association prize. His novels have been translated into English, French, Macedonian and Russian. The translator of this story, Mihnea Arion, is his son.

MEREDITH BLEVINS is the author of seven novels for Macmillan, and one non-fiction for Rodale. She has a new story in the works and is also a travel writer. Her life has been filled with bold women who turned their backs on the color beige. The Southwest is home for Meredith and her husband, author Win Blevins. For more: www.prowriterstoolbox.com

JACQUI BROWN is a blogger at http://www.frenchvillagediaries.com. A British expat, she has been living in southwest France with her husband Adrian and son Ed since August 2004.

ROBIN BURCELL, New York Times Bestselling author, co-writes the Sam and Remi Fargo Adventures with Clive Cussler. Their latest book, *Wrath of Poseidon*, debuted May 26, 2020. www.RobinBurcell.com

TIM CAHILL is the author of nine books, one of which *National Geographic* named as one of the hundred best adventure travel books ever written. He lives in Montana.

TAFFY CANNON is the Agatha- and Macavity-nominated author of fifteen novels, mostly mysteries; an Academy Award-nominated short film; and SibCare: The Trip You Never Planned to Take. She lives in Southern California. www.TaffyCannon.com

RICHARD CASS is the author of the Elder Darrow jazz mystery series, the story of an alcoholic who buys a dive bar in Boston, hoping it will help him get sober. The first book in the series, *In Solo Time*, won the Maine Literary Sward for Crime Fiction. The fifth title, *Sweetie Bogan's Sorrow*, will be published in September 2020. He's also the author of a book of short stories called *Gleam of Bone*. Cass lives and writes in Cape Elizabeth, ME.

SARAH M. CHEN has published numerous short stories and a children's book. Her noir novella *Cleaning Up Finn* was an Anthony finalist and IPPY Award winner. She is the co-editor, along with E.A. Aymar, of *The Swamp Killers* and *The Night of the Flood*. She's written for the *Los Angeles Review of Books, Intrepid Times, Hapa Mag,* and *P.S. I Love You.*

JOHN CLARK is a retired librarian and active book reviewer with a background in mental health. He gardens and continues to write young adult novels as well as short crime and horror stories. He lives with his wife, a retired professor of nursing, in central Maine.

MATT COYLE is the author of the bestselling Rick Cahill crime series. His books have won the Anthony, Lefty, Ben Franklin Silver, Foreword Reviews Book of the Year Silver, and San Diego Book Awards, and have been nominated for the Macavity and Shamus Awards. Matt hosts the Crime Corner podcast on the Authors on the

Air Global Radio Network and lives in San Diego with his yellow Lab, Angus, where he is writing his eighth crime novel. https://mattcoylebooks.com/

Z.J. CZUPOR lives in Denver with his wife and two rescued collies. He writes a monthly column, The Mystery Minute, for the Rocky Mountain Chapter Mystery Writers of America. They can be found at www.rmmwa.org. Since the coronavirus pandemic started, Z.J. began writing and posting poetry on Facebook in the form of haikus, called "Today's Noir Haiku." Follow the entire thread at www.facebook.com/zjczupor.

J. MADISON DAVIS is the author of eight novels—several of which were nominated for awards and one of which was briefly an e-book best seller. He has also published seven nonfiction books, and dozens of short stories and articles. He was a columnist on international crime writing for World Literature Today for fifteen years, and is a Professor Emeritus of the University of Oklahoma. In the summer of 2008, he was elected the President of the International Association of Crime Writers, and now lives at Lake Monticello, Virginia.

A native of Co. Roscommon, Ireland, EOGHAN EGAN wrote his first story aged nine. A graduate of Maynooth University's Creative Writing Curriculum, Eoghan divides his time between Roscommon, Dublin, and Southern Italy. The first in his trilogy of crime fiction novels, *Hiding in Plain Sight*, was released in January 2020. https://eoghanegan.com/

DAN FESPERMAN'S eleven novels of mystery and suspense have won international acclaim, winning the Dashiell Hammett award in the US and two Dagger awards in the UK. A former foreign correspondent for the *Baltimore Sun*, his travels have taken him to three war zones and more than thirty countries. He grew up in North Carolina, graduated from UNC-Chapel Hill, and now lives in Baltimore.

KATE FLORA is the author of 21 books in fiction, true crime, nonfiction, and short fiction. She's been an editor and a publisher, international president of Sisters in Crime, and a founding member of the New England Crimebake and Maine Crime Wave conferences and runs the Maine Crime Writers blog. She's been a finalist for the Edgar, Anthony, Agatha and Derringer awards, won the Public Safety Writers Award and twice won the Maine Literary Award for Crime Fiction. She's an enthusiastic gardener with a brown thumb and excels at burning rice. Flora divides her time between Maine and Massachusetts and dreams of being a torch singer though she sings like a frog. www.kateclarkflora.com

TAMI HAALAND is the author of three poetry collections, most recently *What Does Not Return*. Her poems have appeared in many periodicals and anthologies, including, Consequence, The American Journal of Poetry, Ascent, The Ecopoetry Anthology, and Healing the Divide. Her work has also been featured on The Slowdown, The Writer's Almanac, Verse Daily, and American Life in Poetry. Haaland lives and teaches in Montana.

NAOMI HIRAHARA is the Edgar Award-winning author of two mystery series set in Southern California. Her Mas Arai series, which features a Hiroshima survivor and Altadena gardener, ended with the publication of Hiroshima Boy in 2018. Her Hawai'I mystery, Iced in Paradise, was released in September 2019. Her new historic stand-alone set in 1944 Chicago, Clark and Division, will be published by Soho Crime in May 2021. A former editor of The Rafu Shimpo newspaper, she has also published noir short stories, middle-grade fiction and nonfiction history books. She was born in Pasadena and lives there today. www.naomihirahara.com

An NPR interviewer aptly described Edgar-Award winning author WENDY HORNSBY as "a genteel college professor by day, and by night a purveyor of murder most foul." Now Professor of History Emeritus, she has abandoned all pretense of gentility in order to purvey stories of foul murder full time. She is the author of fifteen books and many short stories. *A Bouquet of Rue*, (Perseverance Press, April 2019), her most recent Maggie MacGowen mystery, is available now, and her story, "Ten Years, Two Days, and Six Hours," can be found in *Deadly Anniversaries* (Hanover Square Press, April 2020). www.wendyhornsby.com

JODY JAFFE is the author of the Nattie Gold newspaper/horse show mysteries: *Horse of a Different Killer, Chestnut Mare, Beware,* and *In Colt Blood*. She is also the co-author of the novels *Thief of Words* and *Shenandoah Summer*. She and her husband, John Muncie, live on a farm in the Shenandoah Valley with eight horses.

PAUL JEFFCUTT's second collection, *The Skylark's Call,* is forthcoming from Dempsey & Windle; his first, *Latch,* was published by Lagan Press. Recently his poems have appeared in The Honest Ulsterman, Ink, Sweat & Tears, The Interpreter's House, Magma, Orbis, Oxford Poetry, Poetry Ireland Review, Poetry Salzburg Review and Vallum. He lives in Co Down, Northern Ireland. www.pauljeffcutt.net

ALLEN MORRIS JONES is the Spur Award-winning author of the novels *Sweeney on the Rocks, A Bloom of Bones,* and *Last Year's River*, as well as a nonfiction consideration of the ethics of hunting, *A Quiet Place of Violence,* and a children's book, *Montana for Kids: The Story of Our State*. He lives in Bozeman, Montana, with his wife and young son.

TATJANA KRUSE is a mystery writer whose credits include the Sleuth Sisters Konny and Kriemhild, the needleworking Ex-Detective Siggi Seifferheld and the Opera Singer/Private Eye Pauline Miller with her narcoleptic Boston Terrier Radames. In her former life, Tatjana worked as executive assistant, bookseller and literary translator. In her latest (and favorite) incarnation as a mystery novelist, she is a bestselling author and winner of several awards, including the Chandler Society's Marlowe award for Best German Short Story. She lives in the South of Germany. www.tatjanakruse.de

CRAIG LANCASTER was once called "one of the most important writers in Montana," and it wasn't even his mother who said it. (It was David Crisp, the founder and editor of the late, lamented Billings Outpost.) He's written eight published novels, notably the High Plains Book Award-winning 600 Hours of Edward, as well as a collection of short stories. He's a staff editor at the sports journalism site The Athletic and also serves as the design director of and a frequent contributor to Montana Quarterly magazine.. He lives in Billings, Montana, with his wife, novelist Elisa Lorello. www.craig-lancaster.com

Italian author ADRIANA LICIO spent 6 years in her beloved Scotland, and has never recovered. She lives somewhere in the Apennine mountains in southern Italy and whenever she can, rushes to Maratea, the seaside setting of her Italian Village Mystery series, featuring travel writer Giò Brando. When not under lockdown, she also runs her family perfumery shop. https://adrianalicio.com

LISE McCLENDON is the author of 23 novels and numerous short stories. She serves on the faculty of the Jackson Hole Writers Conference and has been a board member of Mystery Writers of America and International Crime Writers Association/North America. She began her career with *The Bluejay Shaman*, set in her home state of Montana, and now writes a series set in France, the **Bennett Sisters Mysteries**. She lives in Montana and California. lisemcclendon.com

MIKE MONSON is the author of the noir/crime novellas *The Scent of New Death, What Happens in Reno*, and *A Killer's Love,* as well as the crime novel *Tussinland.* He is preparing to publish the book, *Ridesharing,* a collection of fictional stories based on his experiences as an Uber/Lyft driver. He has written a feature movie script based on his novella What Happens in Reno, and is working on a script based on The Scent of New Death (retitled for the screen as Revenge Plot).

Also, he is creating scripts for a projected anthology TV series based on the stories in *Ridesharing*. He is a graduate of Chapman University.

DONNA MOORE is the author of two humorous crime fiction novels and several short stories. She is currently undertaking a PhD in Creative Writing, writing three historical crime fiction novellas set between 1870 and 1920. In her day job she works with marginalized and vulnerable women to support them with their literacy. She is also co-host of the CrimeFest crime fiction convention. Oh, and she (reluctantly) knows far too much about ants. She lives in Scotland.

SHARAN NEWMAN is a medieval historian who writes the Catherine Lavender mysteries and also non-fiction. She lives near a village in Ireland with a view of the Shannon Estuary, where people take the supernatural as normal. http://www.sharannewman.com

JIM NISBET has published twenty books: thirteen novels including *Lethal Injection*, a classic roman noir, six volumes of poetry, and a nonfiction title, *Laminating The Conic Frustum*. He is at work on two more novels, a complete translation of Charles Baudelaire's *Les Fleurs du Mal*, and a growing collection of Plague Ditties. He lives in the Bay Area, California. http://noirconeville.com/

GARY PHILLIPS writes anything he can get away with. His latest is a novel wherein real life North Pole explorer Matthew Henson is reimagined as a pulp adventurer in the Indiana Jones mold, set in the Roaring '20s: *Matthew Henson and the Ice Temple of Harlem*. He lives in Los Angeles.

JOHN REMBER lives and writes in the Sawtooth Valley of Idaho. Recurring themes in his writing include the meaning of place, the impact of tourism on the West, and the fragility of industrial civilization. John's latest book, *A Hundred Little Pieces on the End of the World* was published in March 2020 by the University of New Mexico Press.

TRAVIS RICHARDSON has been a finalist and nominee for the Macavity, Anthony, and Derringer short story awards. He has 2 novellas, LOST IN CLOVER and KEEPING THE RECORD. His short story collection, BLOODSHOT AND BRUISED, came out in late 2018. He lives in Los Angeles with his wife and daughter. http://www.tsrichardson.com

A servant to two cats, MERRILEE ROBSON uses the time when the cats are sleeping to write mysteries. Fortunately, cats sleep a lot. Her first novel, *Murder is Uncooperative*, is set in a Vancouver housing co-op. Her short crime fiction has recently appeared in Ellery Queen Mystery Magazine, The People's Friend, Over My Dead Body, Mysteryrat's Maze podcast, Mystery Weekly, and other magazines and anthologies, including the upcoming Malice Domestic 15: Mystery Most Theatrical.. She lives in Vancouver, Canada. www.merrileerobson.ca.

CAITLIN ROTHER is the *New York Times* bestselling author or co-author of 13 books, including DEAD RECKONING, HUNTING CHARLES MANSON, and POISONED LOVE. Coming soon is DEATH ON OCEAN BOULEVARD: Inside the Coronado Mansion Case. She lives in San Diego. https://www.caitlinrother.com

WENDY SALINGER'S memoir *Listen* (Bloomsbury, 2006), was nominated for The Krause Essay Prize. Her book of poetry, *Folly River* (Dutton, 1980), was the winner of the first Open Competition of The National Poetry Series. She lives in New York City where she directs The Walker Literature Project at the 92nd Street Y.

JOHN SHEPPHIRD is a Shamus Award-winning author and writer/director of television movies. Mystery Scene Magazine calls his novel BOTTOM FEEDERS "A fast-paced, fun read that explores a part of the movie business that often gets overlooked... from 'Action!' to 'Cut' it's a pleasure to read." He lives in California. johnshepphird.com

KEITH SNYDER'S short story, "Blue Skies," appears in issue 5 of *Black Cat Mystery Magazine*.

From New York, GERALD SO is editor of The Five-Two weekly crime poetry site, new every Monday at http://poemsoncrime.blogspot.com. Follow him on Twitter @g_so.

MARIAN McMAHON STANLEY enjoyed a long international career and, most recently, a second at a large urban university. A dual citizen of the United States and Ireland, she lives outside Boston with her husband Bill and a Westie named Archie. She is the author of two Rosaria O'Reilly mysteries *The Immaculate* and *Buried Troubles*, as well as a number of short stories.

PIET TEIGELER was born in 1936 in Antwerp, Belgium. After retiring from journalism, he published 17 mystery novels in Dutch. Four were nominated for the Hercule Poirot Prize which he won in 2000 for '*The Black Death*'. He was worldwide president of AIEP-IACW from 2003 until 2007 and has lived in Spain since 1998.

————

Thanks For Helping !!

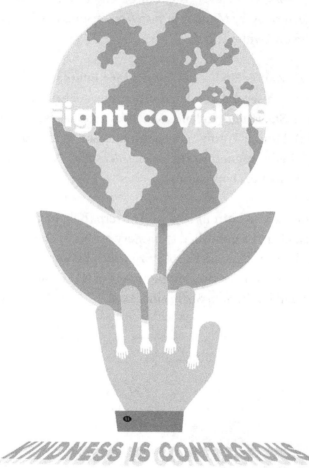

Special thanks to ADITI JAIN and all the UN Covid-19 Response Team Creative
Content artists ♥

See all the artworks at https://unitednations.
talenthouse.com/artworks/

AFTERWORD

Thank you for your purchase of this anthology. We, the editors and contributors, have all donated our time and talent to make this book possible. Did it keep us sane during these crazy times? Time will tell. But it made us feel like we are contributing to the greater good, to humanity's health and well-being, and that is never a bad thing.

All profits from the publication of this book will be donated to charities to be announced at the end of 2020. Please feel free to chime in with your suggestions for beneficiaries, whether in global health, solidarity, law and justice, or artists and writers. All of these are excellent causes and in need of public support.

Please leave a review at the site where you purchased the book. This one small act of support may encourage others to buy the book and thus increase our donations.

Thank you.

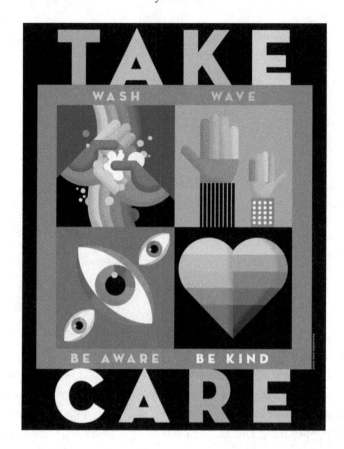